A MIND APART

A Mind Apart

Understanding Children with Autism and Asperger Syndrome

PETER SZATMARI

THE GUILFORD PRESS
New York · London

To Dyanne, Kathryn, Claire, and Josie

The more complete the joy of loving is.

—DANTE, *The Divine Comedy*

Library of Congress Cataloging-in-Publication Data

Szatmari, Peter.
A mind apart : understanding children with autism and Asperger
syndrome / by Peter Szatmari.
    p. cm.
Includes bibliographical references and index.
  ISBN 1-57230-544-4 (pbk.) — ISBN 1-59385-030-1 (hardcover)
  1. Autism in children. 2. Autistic children—Case studies. 3.
Developmental disabilities. I. Title.
  RJ506.A9S99 2004
  618.92'8909—dc22

                                            2003026345

Contents

Contents

Preface

"It all depends on the way you see things," said the woman on the other side of the little table in my office. "Once you understand how they think and see the world, what can seem like a disability one day can be a talent, or a gift, on another."

The words struck me like a thunderbolt. The way you "see" things? That there were different ways of viewing disability—including, in some circumstances, as a gift—was something I had known on an intellectual level for a long time in my work with children with autism spectrum disorders (ASDs). But somehow I had never truly appreciated the concept until it was uttered by Marsha, the mother of Chris, a teenager with Asperger syndrome. What a difference it would make, I realized, to understand how kids with ASDs "see" the world and how that would change the way we "see" the kids. This turned out to be the key to what I had been looking for, the link to tie together the various strands I had been thinking about and trying to articulate in explaining the science of autism to parents of children with these perplexing disorders. It was hearing these words that helped me write this book.

Marsha had spoken these words in response to a question I had asked: What had helped her cope with the stress of raising a child with ASD? How had she survived those years when Chris was having difficulty in school, when he was not quite living up to family and school "expectations," when so many people, trying to be helpful, could not resist remarking that he was not quite "normal" (whatever that is)? The extra time Marsha had to spend with Chris was a real burden on the rest of the family. She elaborated that once she and her husband were able to understand him, what made him think and feel in a different way, life became ever so much easier. Now it seemed like living with an adolescent with ASD was no more difficult than living with any teenager (admittedly not an easy task at the best of times!). Marsha had learned to look into the inner world of her child's mind, and that view and perspective had made a major difference to her, to her family, and, most important of all, to Chris himself.

I have seen parents experience much confusion and anxiety upon hearing terms such as "impairments in reciprocal social interaction" and "stereotyped behaviors" when what they are trying to deal with is a child who ignores their requests to play or rocks himself repetitively or lines up little figures across the floor over and over again. I have seen how parents react when they realize their young child doesn't cuddle with them or does not run to greet them when they've been out all day. It must seem impossible to understand this behavior; to have a child who appears capable of doing incredible jigsaw puzzles one day, of being able to program the most complicated video machine on another day, but who doesn't speak at all, who does not communicate the simplest phrase. In this book, I have tried to explore these and other behaviors through stories that illustrate how understanding individual children can help parents enter the inner world of their children, can understand where these behaviors come from, and then can implement intervention and treatment strategies that make a true and lasting difference.

It is important to focus on real experiences as a way of understanding, but communicating that experience can be a daunting and difficult task. The difficulty surely lies in the fact that children with ASD use a secret language to communicate; they see the world from a unique perspective and experience themselves and others differently. They live in a mysterious world of direct perception and immediacy; they see a world without metaphors. They are "a mind apart," but at the same time they are still children for all that. This difference in perspectives is hard for parents and professionals to understand at first glance. It means traveling to a "foreign country" and learning a new language. The inescapable difficulties in communication often lead to stereotyping, misunderstanding, and stigma. Marsha experienced the hostility and rejection of uncles and aunts who could not tolerate Chris's disruptive behavior at family gatherings, and she experienced the disapproving looks of complete strangers in the grocery store who watched him become upset because he could not have a specific brand of cereal. She could tell they thought she was a terrible mother who spoiled her child. Greater understanding of these disruptive and perplexing behaviors is possible once we can see the world through the child's eyes. That perspective can lead to a better and more respectful approach to treatment and eventually to a better outcome in the future.

Without a name for their child's baffling behavior, parents fear the unknown and look ahead with dread and apprehension. But truly understanding the disease, the illness and the predicaments of the child with an ASD, will go a long way toward fending off the despair that many families experience, particularly at the beginning of their journey as they seek a diagnosis and embark on a treatment plan. Coming to understand a child with autism or Asperger syndrome means learning that a behavior interpreted one way, based on our intuition and experience with human nature, must instead be viewed in an entirely different way, as a product of the different thought processes that are characteristic of these children.

This book is structured as a collection of clinical tales that illustrates imaginatively the lives of children with autism and Asperger syndrome. You may recognize in them some of the confusing behaviors you see in your own child. You may also recognize, in the parents depicted, some of the experiences that your own family has gone through in trying to obtain information about diagnosis, outcome, and treatment. This book is an attempt to lay out the foundations for understanding the minds of children with ASDs—how they think, how they perceive things, what they can and can't do as a result. Its goal is also to change the way we "see" these children. My hope is that by reading this book, parents—and others who work with these children, in schools and elsewhere—will also arrive at the understanding that Marsha developed over time, but do so at an earlier stage. For, in the end, perhaps the most powerful treatment we have at our disposal is knowledge, knowledge that clears away misunderstanding, restores hope and a sense of control over one's destiny. I hope it will become possible to develop a stronger bond with your child, as well as help him or her reach for the best chance at a happy life. Coming to understand the way the child thinks and feels and how that translates to often baffling, sometimes disturbing behavior will do away with the many obstacles that appear to stand in the way of both rewarding parent–child relationships and effective interventions. Then children with ASD become children just like other, more typical children.

My clinical practice over the last twenty years has been devoted ex-

clusively to diagnosing and assessing children with ASD and to helping
parents, teachers, and the children themselves cope, come to terms
with, and sometimes even celebrate, the predicaments associated with
ASD. My frustration at not knowing enough has also encouraged me to
do research into the causes of autism, into what Asperger syndrome
looks like, how it differs from autism, and how children with ASD
change over time through adolescence and into adulthood. I have seen
some individuals with ASD become mature and articulate adults and
have seen others struggle with significant and heart-wrenching difficulties. When I look back over those twenty years and try to single out the
most important ingredient associated with a successful outcome, I come
back, time and again, to the importance of having a family or a teacher
understand what it's like to be inside the mind of a child with ASD. For
understanding leads to a sense of empathy with the child, and that leads
to the development of a special relationship without which any intervention program is bound to fail.

To feel this empathy, parents need a passport to that foreign country of "a mind apart"; they need a code book to understand the puzzling
and contradictory language of their child. Realizing that one's child has
autism or Asperger syndrome or pervasive developmental disorder not
otherwise specified (PDDNOS) forces a confrontation with the apparent
cruelty of biology and the loss of the perfect child, a dream shared by all
prospective parents. That inevitably leads to grief, unhappiness, and a
sense of anxiety about the future. Coming to terms with this grief is
possible, however, and, in my experience, involves seeing the world as
their child experiences it, a process that can take many years. The confusion and pain parents feel at first (and intermittently thereafter) is the
result of not understanding this experience and its changing manifestations. I hope this book will change that.

It takes an imaginative leap to understand children with ASD,
which is why the clinical tales I have told are presented imaginatively.
That does not mean, however, that the information embedded in the
tales is not "evidence-based." The stories, in fact, are used to illustrate
what science has been able to tell us about autism and Asperger syndrome according to the "best available evidence." These tales are not
meant to be evidence, as are the so-called case histories that now have a
bad reputation in the biomedical literature, but to communicate the evidence in a valid and accurate way.

Using imagination to explain science may seem like a contradiction
in terms. Science and the imagination are, after all, at the opposite ends

of public consciousness (although this was not always true throughout history) and are often seen to be in conflict. But this is a shortsighted view. Many now recognize that, with the developments in science in the last century, true science cannot be conducted without a vivid imagination. It is the imagination that is used to build models of what we know, a way of tying together the facts into a narrative that makes sense. In an interview sometime before he died, the writer Vladimir Nabokov (who was an expert on the classification of butterflies) said, "There is no science without fancy and no art without facts."

The goal of this book, therefore, is to supply the imagination that goes along with the science. This is more critical in autism perhaps than in other medical conditions since the ASDs are so mysterious, the behaviors seemingly so inexplicable. It takes a feat of imagination to leap across the boundary of our mind to the mind of the child with autism. If it takes imagination to understand, perhaps the best way to convey that is through the medium of stories and personal narrative. I am grateful to the families I have known for allowing me to use their stories— stories that unfolded in their telling over the last twenty years—in the hopes that others may benefit. These stories were inspired by their real experiences, but to protect confidentiality, I have obviously changed details, removed all identifying information, and obtained consent from people who might be identified. The generosity of families that care for children with ASD has never ceased to amaze me, and if this book does some good, then that is my true thanks.

Is it too much to imagine a future where there are enough resources for children with ASD to receive timely and cost-effective services in hospitals, community agencies, and schools? A future where they are not marginalized but instead are valued and loved by all who care for them and teach them? If this book helps in a small way toward that future, I will have paid my debt to Marsha, who taught me "it's all in the way you see things."

Acknowledgments

Many people have hovered over my shoulder as I was hunched over the keyboard writing these chapters. My friends and colleagues in the Offord Centre for Child Studies gave me lots of encouragement and constructive criticism as I tried to present the scientific evidence. Much of what I have learned came from working with a gifted group of clinicians dedicated to implementing evidence-based service plans for children with autism spectrum disorders. Lorrie Cheevers, Sue Honeyman, Leslie France, Gary Tweedie, Jane Brander, Steven Fraser, Kathy Pierce, and Lorna Colli have all taught me an enormous amount about children with autism and how their families cope with the disorder. Their practical tips and advice on how to implement treatment programs into the busy schedules of parents' lives was invaluable. I have also benefited enormously from other colleagues associated with the team, including Bill Mahoney, Jane Summers, and Jo-Ann Reitzel, who have shared with me their many insights and perspectives. I owe a great deal to my research collaborators, especially Susan Bryson and Lonnie Zwaigenbaum, with whom I have worked so productively over many years. I owe Susan a great deal for her insight, good humor, support, and constructive criticism over the roughly twenty years that we have worked together. Other research colleagues with whom I have benefited enormously include Jeremy Goldberg, Michel Maziade, Roberta Palmour, Marc-Andre Roy, Chantal Merette, Steve Scherer, Andrew Paterson, John Vincent, Isabel Smith, and Wendy Roberts. Jessica DeVilliers and Jonathan Fine provided me with much of the thinking in Chapter 6. It was the opportunity to bounce ideas off all these colleagues that led to much of the research with which I have been involved over the last two decades. My research team, which includes Ann Thompson, Liezanne Vaccarella, Christina Strawbridge, Trish Colton, Sherry Cecil, Stelios Georgiades, and Bev DaSilva, as well as those who have worked with us over the years, have always been extremely productive and supportive in bringing to fruition the many (sometimes half-cocked) research ideas we have dreamed up. They have worked long hours, often in difficult situations and weather, to collect the highest-quality data and have been active collaborators and colleagues. Joan Whitehouse, who is like a rock in the office, has often been the only sane voice in the work environment, and to her I owe a substantial debt.

I have been extremely fortunate in working with major figures in the field of child psychiatry, all of whom have influenced me enormously and have shaped my sensibilities. David Taylor is the reason I am a child psychiatrist, and it is he who has served as my role model as a communicator. His mark is on every page of this book. Dan Offord has taught me so much about research that I will never be able to thank him enough. Marshall Bush Jones has been not only a mentor, but also a colleague and valued friend with whom my research has been most closely identified. Our conversations (usually on a Friday afternoon) have always been a great delight and a source of inspiration for me. I want to thank Rick Ludkin, my kayaking buddy, who has carefully read over each chapter of this book and has made many constructive and informative criticisms. I can only repay him by trying to paddle harder! McMaster University and the Department of Psychiatry have always supported my aspirations and gave me the leeway to write a book like this. I also want to acknowledge the Ontario Mental Health Foundation, the National Alliance for Autism Research, the Canadian Institutes of Health Research, and the Chedoke Health Corporation for their ongoing support of our research efforts over the years. Without this support, the creation of new knowledge would have been impossible and the impetus to disseminate these evidence-based stories would not have occurred.

Kathryn Moore of The Guilford Press had the audacity to support me when I told her that I wanted to write a different kind of book about autism. Most publishers would have looked at me askance, but Kathryn had no hesitation in agreeing. She put me in touch with my editor, Chris Benton, who so often saved me from myself and my tendency toward solipsism. She never said how difficult it must be to take my sometimes tortured sentences and turn them into plain English. For that, and her always astute insights, I am deeply grateful.

My three children—Kathryn, Claire, and Josie—always made me laugh and made sure that I remembered what was important in life. My mother taught me early on the value of art and was so instrumental in stimulating my interest in Asperger syndrome by translating Hans Asperger's paper. My wife, Dyanne, my best friend and closest confidante, inspired whatever beauty and wisdom there is in this book.

Although many people hovered with me over the keyboard and were vocal in their suggestions and criticisms over the years, I take full responsibility for any omissions and errors in presentation. The evidence always changes, and I have done my best to keep up. As Chekhov once said to a reader who asked him the meaning of a short story, "Everyone writes as best he can. I would like to go to heaven, but I haven't the strength."

Chapter 1

Stephen
The Eccentric Entomologist

I sit and watch Stephen play in the afternoon sun outside my window. He is nine years old. I have not seen him for some time, and I'm surprised at how much he's grown. It's a warm day in December, but it feels more like spring as an early snowfall melts on the lawn. I work at an old hospital that used to be a tuberculosis sanatorium, and the maintenance staff are putting up the Christmas lights on a very tall pine tree, as they have done every December for many years. Stephen runs around the path in circles, paying no attention to the lights going up. His mother keeps a slightly anxious eye on him, as do the gentlemen working on the tree. When it's time for me to greet him, he clumps up the stairs, too heavily for so slight a boy. He announces in a loud voice, "I catch wasps!"

"Do you?" I reply, feeling rather taken aback. "That must be dangerous."

But he does not answer. He has a messy crop of blonde hair as well as lots of freckles, and he darts around my office almost like a bird, checking out the toys, the books, and the papers on my crowded desk.

He casts an anxious eye back at me and says, "I don't want to grow up!"

I nod sympathetically and try to inquire why, but again he does not answer. He would rather talk about wasps, which are his passion. He tells me all about the different kinds of wasps that exist in the world, how he has them encased in epoxy at home and how mad they get when he captures them.

1

"Why do you like wasps so much?" I ask.

"I like the sound they make and how their legs hang when they fly."

How their legs hang? I have never noticed the legs of a wasp, when they fly or otherwise. What is there to like about the sound and their legs?

*   *   *

What indeed? This book is about people with autism, Asperger syndrome (AS), and pervasive developmental disorder not otherwise specified (PDDNOS), three common and important forms of autism spectrum disorder (ASD). It is about the sound wasps make and how their legs hang in the air when they fly. Children and adults with ASD have behaviors that professionals characterize as obsessions, preoccupations, rituals, resistance to change, and self-stimulation. But instead parents might see a young boy with an excessive fascination with wasps, a child who insists on keeping all the doors on the second floor of her house open (even the one to her parents' bedroom), or a boy who gets terribly upset if the blanket on his bed is changed or the wrong cup is placed by his plate at breakfast. People with these types of disorder also typically have trouble communicating with adults and children and experience difficulties with relationships in general. In conversation, they may go off on tangents, ask the same question over and over again, even if they know the answer, or talk only about wasps or their particular, often rather eccentric, passion. Parents and other family members know that these are the often debilitating symptoms of a terrible disorder that strikes at the heart of childhood. A thousand times every day, parents feel as if they will never understand what goes on in the mind of their child, that they will never find a common ground with other people who do not have a child with one of these disorders. The simple task of shopping for groceries can become a nightmare as perfect strangers stare at them and pass judgment on their parenting skills.

In this book, I hope to convey to parents and professionals another context: how the world is perceived by children with ASD. In turn, I hope this will change our perception of the children themselves. Behaviors like Stephen's can also be seen as passions that teach us about the world and how it looks and sounds. By unraveling one mystery, I hope to reveal another, more fundamental, one. And that is that children and adults with ASD live in a concrete world, palpable and immediate, a world without metaphors. Theirs is a world of detail and of infinite variety. It is a visual world built of images, not language. Feelings, emotions, and personal relationships do not have the same value for them as they do for us and for other, typical, children. It can be terrifying and confusing to live in such a world, and it is true that the opportunities for growth and development are often limiting. But the way these children perceive the world can change and transform the way we see the world and make it a more magical place, full of wonder and variety. Children with ASD can teach us about the infinite variety of sameness, and, in seeing their diversity, we realize that there is a sameness to us all. Once we appreciate this, our attempts to help children with ASD accommodate to our world can be more successful and perhaps accomplished without the loss of their special gifts.

* * *

Stephen has been interested in wasps for several years. This is not just a passing fancy or a hobby that he finds amusing or that fills in the time between episodes of his favorite TV shows. He is obsessed with wasps, passionate about them. He talks about them all the time, with his teachers, his parents, and grandparents, even with complete strangers. If people show little interest, he chatters on, unaware of the boredom or frustration experienced by his listener. In the summer, he only wants to go to the park or the garden center to chase wasps around the plants and bushes and try to catch them. If, for some reason, his parents cannot take him there, he becomes very upset. Of course it's difficult for him to have a friend over to play since other children are afraid of wasps and do not want to be stung. Stephen has been bitten several times, but this in no way diminishes his enthusiasm. He catches wasps in a bottle and then releases them in his bedroom and enjoys watching them fly around the room, listening to the sound their legs make as they fly through the air, as I now learn. During winter, when the wasps go into hibernation, he spends hours in his room, poring over his collection of wasps encased in epoxy.

At first Stephen's parents were completely bewildered by his interest in wasps and not a little upset. After all, nine-year-old boys should be interested in sports, in toys that shoot and dart about. How could anybody find wasps enchanting? But now they find Stephen's interest charming. They too have acquired a detailed knowledge of the wasp's habits and lifespan. The four of us sit and talk about wasps as if we are all entomologists attending some esoteric conference about the mating habits of the yellow jacket. Stephen's disability has transformed us all; me for a moment, his parents for a lifetime.

In many respects, Stephen's story is quite typical for a child with autism. His parents first became concerned with his development when he reached age one and was not yet crawling. They also noticed that, compared to his older sister, Stephen was very clingy and could amuse himself for long periods of time by making humming noises. His parents took him to see a pediatrician, and this led to several assessments that finally, at age three, produced a diagnosis of autism. The time between that first visit to the pediatrician and the official diagnosis was very stressful for the family, and they became increasingly alarmed about Stephen's development. Living without a diagnosis was very difficult. In such circumstances parents tend to blame themselves for their child's delays in development, and these recriminations become ever more strident, as the time taken to arrive at an answer lengthens.

When I saw him at three years, Stephen spoke a few words but used them only occasionally to label objects. More often, he would yell, cry, or protest. He did not compensate for his lack of speech by pointing at things, gesturing, or nodding and shaking his head to indicate "yes" or "no." Although, for the most part, he seemed to be happy, he would not smile back at his parents when they smiled at him. When his father came home from work, Stephen would not run to the door to greet him but would jump up and down and flap his arms instead. He would not hug or kiss his parents and did not enjoy cuddling. He tolerated being held by them but generally did not reciprocate their affection. He would often run his hands through his mother's hair and then sniff them. In general, he would not ask his parents to join his play activities and did not direct their attention to toys with which he was playing. If he hurt himself, he would not come for comfort and would not offer comfort to his older sister if he saw that she was crying.

He loved to play with balls, though. He would spin them, throw them, bounce them off the ground, and line them up. He liked to carry a globe around with him all the time so that he could look through the hole from one end to the other. He also enjoyed watching water go down the toilet and playing with cars, but only if they went around in circles. He became particularly excited if the antennae wobbled. He also loved to watch ants travel across the pavement and to drop sand on his balloons or pour water over them. Even though he experienced considerable pleasure from these activities, he would not share his enjoyment with others; he would not have his parents come and watch him move the cars or have them look at how happy he was. He would play with other children, but only if the games involved balls or playing tag. Left to his own devices, he would usually play with a ball, wiggle the antennae on toy cars, or lie happily in bed making humming noises to himself.

Stephen had one ritual, and that was to insist that his parents give him a hug before he entered the kitchen for breakfast. If for some reason this was not possible, he would become very upset and could not be comforted or reassured. He would also become distraught if one of his balloons made a loud noise when the air escaped. He was particularly afraid of the balloon flying around the room.

At age three Stephen began to attend a community school four mornings a week. There, he had an opportunity to be with typical children in a structured situation and with a special teacher who worked with him very closely. She had experience in working with children with ASD and was aware of the many strategies that are effective in promoting social interaction and communication. (Sources of information on such strategies are listed at the back of this book and are referred to throughout the book.) A year later, he was talking in short sentences and even asking questions. He now enjoyed being with the other children and would even initiate some rough-and-tumble play with them, although very little of his play consisted of sharing or turn taking. There was also still no evidence of pretend play with his cars or action figures, and he started to flap his arms and walk on his toes when excited. He continued to be fascinated by water and by balloons, but now he added an interest in the moon and in vacuum cleaners to his list of fascinations.

Obviously, Stephen's interest in wasps was just one of a long line of special interests and preoccupations. The first consisted of very simple visual stimuli: water going down the toilet, looking through holes, dropping sand, wobbling antennae, and bouncing balls. As he matured, the interests become more complex (the moon, vacuum cleaners, and wasps), but all shared the quality of variation in shape, movement, color, and pattern. Sometimes the visual stimuli were accompanied by sounds—simple humming noises and the sounds wasps make when they fly. Shapes, movement, patterns, and sounds never lost their immediacy and their magnetic appeal for him. Stephen, it seemed, had a gift for not being easily bored by the simple things of life.

* * *

Many people think of the child with autism as someone who is totally mute, completely self-absorbed, and who sits in a corner and rocks all day. Other common misperceptions are that people with autism are extremely violent and aggressive, capable of the most horrific forms of self-mutilation, such as gouging out their eyes or banging their heads. Stephen shows none of these behaviors or attributes; he is talkative and gentle, and he is engaged in the world, except he sees the world from his own perspective. He is completely endearing and charming in an eccentric way. The child with autism as popularized by the media and television shows is nowadays quite rare. Such individuals were much more common when disabled children were removed from their homes and placed in large institutions with little stimulation or opportunities for useful activities and social interaction.

There is, in fact, enormous variety in how autism presents in individual children. While it's true that many people with autism are not capable of functionally useful language, a substantial proportion, perhaps more than fifty percent, are able to use language, at least to have their essential needs met. It is also true that the vast majority of children with autism do interact socially with other children and with adults but do so in a limited, unusual, or fixed fashion. It is the *quality* of their social interaction that sets children with autism apart from other individuals, not whether they do or do not interact. There is also enormous variation in their cognitive abilities. Some children with autism are able to perform only rudimentary arithmetical operations, and some will never learn to read. Others, however, are able to perform the most astonishing mathematical calculations, or are able to identify the day of the week on which any individual is born in any year. And some have an amazing capacity to read at an early age or have an encyclopedic knowledge of specific topics.

In spite of this enormous diversity, there are three key features that characterize all children with autism, AS, and PDDNOS. These are impairments in reciprocal social interaction, impairments in verbal and nonverbal communication, and a preference for repetitive, solitary, and stereotyped interests or activities. In other words, children and adults with any form of ASD demonstrate a difficulty (1) in building social relationships and (2) in communicating through words, gestures, and facial expression, and they all (3) spend their spare time doing puzzles, watching things, collecting things, or being fascinated with shiny objects or specific topics and the like. These three general characteristics make up the autistic triad as articulated first by Lorna Wing, and the triad underlies the astonishing number of behaviors that a child with autism may show at one time or another. It is also important to appreciate, as illustrated by Stephen's story, that the symptoms and behaviors vary with the developmental level and age of the individual and can change dramatically over time. But these changes are usually a variation on the theme already contained in the notion of the autistic triad.

For parents, it's the impairments in social reciprocity that most clearly define the predicament of the child and family. The simplest social interactions between parent and child and between siblings, which other families may take for granted, can be extremely difficult for a child with ASD. The rapid building of satisfying relationships, often the most natural thing in the world for most families, becomes instead an arduous task for families where a child has autism. Many of the children limit their social overtures to those required to get their personal needs met, such as asking for help with a toy or getting food from the fridge. The children who do approach their parents for more intricate social interaction often do so for physical games such as tickling, wrestling, and tag, which are enjoyed not so much for the social enjoyment as for the physical sensations these activities evoke. Other children with autism show *too much* social initiative, acting overly friendly with strangers or hugging other children or adults when it's inappropriate. When they do make friends, play activities are often limited to those that fascinate the child with autism, whether it's playing with computer games, watching TV, or setting up scenarios with action figures. Parents may point to these relationships as a sign that their child's social impairment is not all that bad. But it's important to understand that even if the child likes to wrestle with his big brother and will play with miniature cars for hours on end with the little boy next door, the social world does not have the same value and meaning for the child with autism as it does for other, typically developing children, and this difference will affect other areas of the child's life as he grows up. For typical children, social praise, subtle threats such as raising an eyebrow or using a firm tone of voice, and social approbation are powerful learning tools precisely because social interaction holds such high value for them. For the child with ASD, the value of social interaction does not carry the same weight or meaning. As the children mature, these impairments in understanding social interaction evolve into difficulties with empathy and understanding the motivations, beliefs, and feelings of others and themselves. They lack a theory, or an intuitive understanding, of other people's minds and of their own minds. For example, it might be all right for a child with AS to run his fingers through his mother's hair, but it would be quite inappropriate to do that to a complete stranger in the grocery store. No doubt the stranger would be mortified, but the child with AS might not have a clue how that person would feel. Teenagers with AS have a terrible time in high school as they try desperately to understand the ins and outs of dating. The idea that first you have to be "friends" with a girl before she can be a "girlfriend" is often too much for them. It is the subtlety of language and social nuance that proves elusive and confounds their attempts at making deep and meaningful friendships based on mutual understanding.

Difficulties in communication also place a demand on their ability to navigate the social world. Even if they were to develop vocabulary and a mastery of grammar at the same pace as typical children, children with autism and AS do not use language on a day-to-day basis to negotiate the social world, to build bridges between themselves and other people. Their speech is often limited to everyday tasks and to simple requests to meet their own needs: asking for help, going to the park, finding certain favorite toys and objects such as stones, hubcaps, and maps. If they lack speech, they do not substitute nonverbal means of communication as do children who only have simple delays in speech, who can point and gesture in ways that their parents find easy to interpret. The parents of children with autism often have to guess what the meaning of a behavior might be. A familiar story is that a child will pull his parents by the hand to the fridge, indicating a desire for food. A mother will stand in front of the open fridge, getting out different food items, because she has no clue what treat the child is actually requesting. The only way of knowing that the right item has been selected is that the child suddenly stops crying and trots off to the family room with his Popsicle or chocolate milk firmly in hand, without a glance back at the exasperated parent who never learned the knack of reading minds.

Those children with autism who do develop fluent language will often talk incessantly about their favorite subjects—TV shows, sports statistics, the characteristics of subway trains, the sound of thunder, flags of the world, wasps, and so on. Their conversation is rarely recipocal in the sense that it builds on a listener's contribution to the conversation or refers to events or experiences taking place in the wider social context. Their references are mostly to the physical world and tied to their immediate surroundings.

In some cases, it may not be so much that children with autism are unable to speak as it is that they do not have the motivation to use their communication skills for social interaction. A story in the life of one particular boy illustrates this point quite well. Gavin was nineteen years old and was severely affected with autism. While he spoke a few words as a toddler, by the time he was five he was totally mute and did not communicate with words. Instead he used a variety of nonverbal ways of communicating, such as pulling his parents by the hand, pointing, or simply protesting. As he matured, he ignored others altogether and looked after himself quite independently. One of his favorite activities as a teenager was to go on family outings to an amusement park filled with wild and exotic animals from Africa. Gavin particularly enjoyed watching the monkeys dance around the car as the family drove through the park. On this Sunday afternoon, Gavin was sitting in the back seat of the car while his parents were in the front. His parents noticed a very large giraffe approaching the car, but they were distracted by a large troupe of monkeys cavorting playfully on the hood. All of a sudden, they heard a loud voice from the back seat shout, "Get that thing out of here!" The giraffe had put its head through the back window of the car, and Gavin was so frightened that he spoke for the first time in years. He had not said a word for fourteen years, and to his parents' knowledge, never said another word after that one, perfectly formed, articulate emphatic sentence. Once the motivation to communicate was there, Gavin was able to speak; however, in the normal circumstances of everyday life, there was not enough motivation to communicate. Whether other children with autism who are mute are capable of such perfect speech under the right circumstances is not known, but we have learned that motivation plays a major role in speech therapy.

The third characteristic feature of children with autism and AS is the preference for repetitive, solitary, stereotyped behaviors, activities, or interests. What does have value and meaning for children with ASD is the world of concrete sensation. Their play activities repeatedly recreate situations that evoke sensory stimulation in one form or another. There is an almost endless variety of objects that can catch the interest of the child. These may involve spinning wheels, flashing lights, water dripping into the sink, bubbles, kites flying in the wind, letters, numbers—the list is endless. As the children mature, concrete facts or esoteric bits of knowledge can replace more immediate sensory stimulation, so that flags of the world, bus timetables, plumbing, computer programming, or drafting can replace these more immediate sensory experiences. Nevertheless, the essential feature is that these activities are highly concrete, are not psychological in nature but are more like systematizing, are pursued independently of other people, and can provide amusement and fun for the child for hours on end.

Rituals and resistance to change are other manifestations of this third construct that can often cause considerable difficulty for the family. Many children with autism find it very difficult to tolerate trivial changes in their personal environment or routine. Major changes such as moving house or going to a different school may be accepted with equanimity, but changing the furniture in the living room or the blankets on the bed can cause an uproar. Rituals are fixed patterns of behavior that serve no obvious function and that have to be performed in a specific sequence. They are difficult to distinguish from resistance to change, but some examples include keeping all the doors open in the house, touching the bush at the end of the veranda before entering the house, placing one's kitchen utensils in a certain pattern, getting dressed in a particular order. Children with autism have to perform rituals such as these or else their anxiety escalates and aggressive, noncompliant behavior may occur in response to the interruption of that fixed sequence of activities.

Stephen exhibited many aspects of the autistic triad, and these changed with his development and maturity. His social overture to me at our appointment was unusual and reflected his one-sided interests. His communication was characterized by comments that seemingly came out of nowhere but in fact were motivated by his own eccentric interests. Early on, he did not use gestures or facial expression to add emphasis to his words, and to this day he often carries a fixed smile as he stares intently at another person, questioning whether any wasp's nests could be seen in their garden. No? Perhaps there was one hidden by the branches of a bush? Did any wasps visit the compost heap? Or the apples that fell from the tree in the orchard of the conservation park? And so on, and on, as the eyes of the listener glaze over in the face of this relentless onslaught of intense and passionate observation and inquiry.

*   *   *

The classification of autism and the other ASDs has had a long and mostly confusing history. While the term "autism" is well known, the term "pervasive developmental disorder (PDD)" is of more recent origin, and its meaning is not immediately obvious. PDD is the term that is used in the official diagnostic manuals published by the American Psychiatric Association and the World Health Organization. It is true that the disorder is pervasive, insofar as the autistic triad pervades all aspects *PDD* of a child's life. It is also developmental in the sense that it first appears within the first two or three years of life and the manifestations change over time. In addition to autism, other types of PDD have been identified as well. These include Asperger syndrome, atypical autism or PDDNOS, disintegrative disorder of childhood, and Rett's disorder. As these terms are relatively new, the clinical features that distinguish these types of PDD from autism have not yet been established firmly. Moreover, whether these different subtypes are caused by different processes is a subject of considerable current controversy. Nevertheless, it's useful to think of a spectrum of disorders with autism at one end and Asperger syndrome at the other. Indeed, some people prefer the term "autism spectrum disorders (ASD)" rather than PDD. The term PDD implies different disorders that vary in several ways, whereas the term ASD implies a spectrum of related conditions that vary only by severity of symptoms. There are not yet enough research data to choose which of these two terms might be the most appropriate, and enormous confusion about their use exists among both professionals and parents. Many people use the term PDD for a disorder that is different from autism: "My child was given a diagnosis of PDD, not autism," many parents will say. Since PDD is a general category and autism a more specific example of a PDD, this usage is not strictly correct but is certainly understandable. The problem is that the diagnostic criteria for autism have changed dramatically over the last twenty years, and the results of this research have often been confusing, contradictory, and controversial.

Autism was originally described by Leo Kanner. He was the first academic child psychiatrist in the United States and wrote the first textbook on the subject. In a classic paper published in 1943, he described eleven children who tended to be aloof, had unusual patterns of communication, and were very insistent that things in their environment stay the same. He used the term "infantile autism" to describe these children, and the preceding list of characteristics guided the diagnosis.

Over the years, these criteria were refined and basically codified in the third edition of the official classification scheme used in North America, the *Diagnostic and Statistical Manual of Mental Disorders* (DSM-III) of the American Psychiatric Association, which appeared in 1980.

But clinicians had also been aware from the beginning that there were many children who were similar to those described by Kanner, though they did not fully meet the description contained in the original paper. Kanner himself was careful to apply the term "infantile autism" to a relatively small group of children. What to call these other children became a problem. At one point, such children were said to be "psychotic" or to have "childhood schizophrenia," a truly unfortunate choice of words. However, work in the United Kingdom by Israel Kolvin, Michael Rutter, and Christopher (Kit) Ounsted correctly pointed out important differences between children with true schizophrenia and those with autism. At roughly the same time, Lorna Wing described in careful detail the larger group of children with autistic-like symptoms and showed how similar they were to those with autism in terms of their social and communication difficulties. This observation led to the concept of a group of disorders called the PDDs, a term that included autism but was not limited to that category.

The problem at that point in the early 1980s was that the criteria for autism derived from the work of Kanner and contained in DSM-III were too narrow and excluded a large number of children who experts believed had autism but for one reason or another did not meet the official criteria. This was an important limitation since diagnostic and treatment resources in many countries depended on a diagnosis of autism (and still do!). In addition, at that point in 1980 there was no evidence that the different PDD subtypes differed from autism in any clinically important way. A decision was made to broaden the criteria for autism to include more children and to collapse all children with PPD but without autism into a category called PDDNOS, or PDD not otherwise specified. This PDDNOS category was intended to include only a small number of children; most children with PDD would have autism. It turned out otherwise. Not only were there many more children who received a diagnosis of autism, but an even larger number received a diagnosis of PDDNOS. This was most unsatisfactory for parents:

"What disorder does my child have, Doctor?"

"He has PDDNOS," the doctor might reply.

"I beg your pardon—what does that mean?"

"It means PDD not otherwise specified."

"I'm sorry, but I still don't understand. Could you be a bit more specific?"

"Well, I can't actually; it's NOS."

Such discussions, which were not uncommon, did not inspire much confidence in the ability of the diagnostician. Soon clinicians dropped the NOS part and started referring to children with PDD as a shorthand and to distinguish them from those with autism. Hence, parents and professionals started to talk about autism and PDD as separate disorders, whereas autism is really a type of PDD. However, very little was known about children with PDD but not autism (a more precise but still clumsy term), and parents searching the library or the Internet found very little. This too led to a lot of confusion, and often parents would ask for a second opinion, or else authorities would not accept PDD as a diagnosis that would allow children to access services.

Another change to the official classification of autism and the other ASDs occurred in 1994, the third change in fifteen years, with the publication of DSM-IV. This time the other PDDs (the PDDNOS group) were more carefully defined in specific categories known as Asperger's disorder, atypical autism, disintegrative disorder, and Rett's disorder. Of these, most is known about Asperger's disorder, and this subtype of PDD is distinguished from autism by an "absence" of clinically significant language and cognitive delay. In other words, such children have many autistic features but do not have global developmental delay and have roughly age-appropriate use of grammar and vocabulary in their speech (this type of ASD is discussed in detail in the other chapters). Children with atypical autism differ from autism in either having fewer symptoms than autism or having a later age at onset. In our research, we have found this category to be a very difficult diagnosis to apply to children consistently. It usually refers to a heterogeneous group of children who either have severe developmental delay and some autistic features, or else to children with very mild early developmental delays who show some symptoms in the repetitive activities domain at an early age but then grow out of them. The trouble is that clinicians all too often cannot agree on whether the child has autism or atypical autism. The current criteria for this subtype are just too vague, and the differences between PDDNOS or atypical autism and typical autism are just too subtle. Children with disintegrative disorder show completely normal development until four years of age, then regress and develop autistic behaviors just like those with autism. It is a very rare subtype of ASD.

Rett's disorder is a very specific condition that occurs only in girls and is characterized by normal development, then a period of slow head growth, loss of speech, hand wringing, and loss of functional hand use. It is so different from autism in its very specific presentation that it should probably not be included as a PDD subtype, particularly since a genetic mutation has now been discovered for Rett's disorder, a mutation that is not seen in the other PDDs.

If this terminology was not meant to be confusing to begin with, it has certainly become so over the years. Part of the problem is that the research has moved very quickly in this field and there is a time lag between the research findings, their publication in the diagnostic manual, and their dissemination and uptake by clinicians and community services. For parents, it is important to separate the wheat from the chaff, as it were, to take away what is well established and what is still a matter of academic debate. What is well established is that there exists a substantial group of children who display the autistic triad as articulated here. As a group, these children have a common clinical presentation and, as far as we can tell, common needs for treatment that focuses on improving skills in socialization, communication, and play, and on eliminating behaviors (like aggression and severe noncompliance) that prevent their inclusion in schools, day care, Cub Scouts, Brownies, and other community activities. The details of treatment will change with the individual characteristics of the child and his or her developmental level, but not the general orientation and approach. Whether or not a child has autism, atypical autism, or Asperger syndrome does not determine the type of treatment required (except that perhaps speech therapy is not as essential in Asperger syndrome since the children have speech). What does matter is whether or not the child has PDD or ASD; that is the crucial diagnosis to make. Perhaps, when more evidence accumulates on subtype-specific treatment, the differentiation between autism and Asperger syndrome will take on more meaning. But that time is not yet upon us. As the chapters that follow show, it's important to get the diagnosis of PDD or ASD early, so that treatment can begin as quickly as possible. In that way, overall outcome is much improved. Too much time spent on deciding what type of ASD a child has or what caused it can lead to unnecessary delay. Heather's story in Chapter 2 recounts a single mother's attempts to come to terms with the diagnosis and what the experience of getting an early diagnosis meant to her.

*   *   *

Susan Sontag has written about how certain diseases that are mysterious and cannot be treated easily have unwittingly and often inappropriately become metaphors for the human condition: the plague, tuberculosis, syphilis, cancer, and, more recently, AIDS. That is because each disease is also an illness, a presentation in the world, and is associated with a predicament that is unique to every affected person. Autism is not so general a metaphor, but what is so tragic is that the impairments in social interaction, in communication, and in play strike at the very heart of what it means to be a child. After all, childhood is about playing with other children, being looked after by adults, learning to talk, and experiencing the pleasures of communicating and exploring the environment in all its diversity. Childhood is about play, fantasy, and creativity within a world of other people. Autism limits the capacity to develop these to the fullest, and the process derails development onto a somewhat different pathway. What I hope to show in this book is that while this derailment is tragic and produces considerable suffering for the family, it also carries with it the capacity to see the world in a way that has its own value. Within the disability, there is a focus on the intimate architecture of the world. There is an innate capacity to see that architecture without the use of metaphors that may obscure what is seen, so that it may be truly appreciated.

Chapter 2

Heather
A World That Revolves
around a Different Axis

Walking through the old neighborhood, you can hear the children's shouts before the schoolyard comes into view. The sounds cut the morning air like metal striking metal. It is a cold November day, and the trees, now bereft of leaves, are stark against the sky. The clouds are a monochrome gray, and no shadows are cast by the movement of the young mother as she walks into town to do her shopping. She thinks about walking past the schoolyard, knowing it's time for recess. Perhaps she can catch a glimpse of her daughter, wave to her, give her a smile and the confidence to work hard in class. Her daughter is six years old, and the separation each morning as Heather is bundled off to school is still difficult. To see her would be a brief moment of pleasure stolen from the inevitable process of growing up and moving on. But she does not want to be a distraction, to pull her daughter away from her play-mates. The mother imagines her daughter skipping rope or playing tag with the kids. Heather is still new to the school, and there have been many problems. Perhaps it's best not to know, to turn down the other corner and go straight into town. But the lure of seeing the tiny figure in the distance is too great, and with a mixture of longing and foreboding the mother turns up the street toward the playground.

Now the children's shouts are louder, almost deafening. There is a long chain-link fence that cuts the schoolyard off from the street, either to protect the children from strangers or, more likely, to try to contain

16

the chaos within the bounds of the school property. The mother stops in front of the fence and searches the yard for a glimpse of her daughter, who is nowhere to be seen. She thinks to herself that these children's games—hopscotch, skipping, tag, and throwing a ball—have been played in one variation or another for centuries. There is a history to these games; they are part of the fabric of childhood. The children are the same; it is the clothes that are different—baseball caps worn backward, high-top sneakers, puffy jackets, trade names displayed proudly as symbols of belonging to a particular culture. These children want to fit in; they want to affiliate with one another, to be a seamless part of their history.

The children are all in groups. Some are walking around and talking, no doubt gossiping about who likes whom, making secret plans, forming new clubs, hatching great schemes for after school, like building forts or climbing trees in the nearby ravine. Some are in larger groups playing games, kicking a ball, or simply running around. The movement is dizzying and confusing, and the mother strains her eyes, searching for her daughter. A group of children are gathered by the outdoor gym equipment. Some are playing on the slide, shrieking with delight, or hanging upside down pretending to be monkeys and making silly sounds. The mother focuses on that scene, knowing her daughter loves to swing and to spin on the tire. But there's no sign of the child who left the apartment this morning and boarded the school bus in her green coat and her cap pulled down firmly over her ears so that she could barely see, all snug against the chill November wind.

The mother becomes anxious and wonders if her daughter was kept inside the school. Was she upset or hurt? Had something gone terribly wrong? It is still so difficult to send Heather off to school and to tolerate this anxiety about an entire day spent beyond her mother's watchful and protective eye. There have been so many phone calls about difficult behavior—biting the teacher, running away, not sitting quietly in circle time, not paying attention, having temper tantrums in assembly. "Please come and pick up your daughter from school as soon as possible," the anonymous voice says on the other end of the telephone. "Something needs to be done," as if her mother should have done that "something" (whatever "that" is) to prevent such behavior from occurring in the first place.

The bell rings, and all the children begin to file in through the doors. The chaos in the schoolyard starts to resolve itself as two orderly lines form at the doors. A ribbon of children funnel through the entrance and are taken in by the warmth of the school. As the yard clears, the mother sees her daughter. Off to one side there is an old oak tree. All the leaves have fallen, and some of the branches are now dead. At the base of the tree, a young girl in a green coat and cap goes round and round the girth, with one hand on the bark and the other hand holding an old tattered bathing suit. The little girl has not heard the bell ring and is oblivious to the children going back into school. Round and round she goes, never taking her eyes off the bark, which holds her attention like a lock, her gaze riveted by the patterns of light and dark and by the texture of the wood as she circles the tree.

The mother starts to feel panic rising from within, afraid that her daughter will be forgotten. The lessons will start without her. Nobody will notice she is not there, sitting in her seat at the back of the class! Another little girl, the last in the line to go in, notices the child going round and round the tree and hesitates as if undecided what to do. She plucks up her courage and runs to the little girl to speak to her, presumably to tell her that the bell has rung and it is time to go in or else they will get into trouble. The teacher will be cross with them. But the mother knows that this threat cannot tear her away from her fascination with the bark. Indeed the daughter does not look at her helpmate, does not respond to her. The endless rivulets of bark, the way they travel into the earth, the brightness of the dirt, the darkness of the spaces between the tree's covering—that is what she sees, and that is what holds her attention.

The friend leaves and goes into the school somewhat confused. The mother's sense of foreboding and dread rises, and she starts to run along the fence that separates her from her daughter. She must get to the entrance and reach her little girl before she gets in trouble again. The fence seems too long, and she runs along the edge shouting "Heather! Heather!" But those shouts, which are now the only sound on the schoolyard that just a moment ago was so noisy, echo off into the gray emptiness of the sky. Finally she reaches the opening in the fence and rushes across the yard to her daughter's side. Out of breath, she asks, "Heather, what are you doing, honey? It's time to go in for school."

Hearing a voice she recognizes, the little girl turns around and looks up at the mother. The corners of her mouth turn up slightly. But there is no exuberant sense of pleasure at this unexpected meeting. It is as if this unnatural moment is the most normal thing in the world. Panting and out of breath, the mother says, "Let's go in." She takes her daughter by the hand, just as she has done every day of Heather's short life. The mother leads her daughter into the school and sends her off in the direction of her classroom. Once again, Heather is out of her mother's protective gaze.

* * *

Some two years later, I went to the school for the annual review of Heather's placement and to make plans for the next year. As I drove into the parking lot and saw the children playing, I was reminded of the story her mother, Janice, had told me the day she found her in the yard after recess all alone. I was curious to see what Heather would be doing today. Perhaps I too could catch a glimpse of her before the meeting. I parked my car and wandered over to the schoolyard to see the children. I noticed the oak tree, but there was no little girl going round and round. I scanned the field to see if I could find her. She should not be too difficult to spot; after all, she would be the one carrying the bathing suit across her arm. She had about five bathing suits that she carried with her everywhere, but the one with the fruit pattern was her favorite. She hated water and refused to go swimming, but she would hang on to those bathing suits for dear life!

I looked for a little girl standing all alone off by herself. There were groups of children on the swings, in the tire, going down the slide, but no Heather. Then I saw her. She was with a group of girls all huddled together, looking at something in Heather's hands. She seemed to be showing them something precious. Perhaps it was some Pokemon figurines that Heather collected. She carried them to school every day in her backpack, and perhaps now she was showing off the newest addition to her collection. Her friends were clearly very impressed, and I imagined that appreciative sounds were made about this character's color or that figure's shape. Heather was clearly proud to be the center of attention and eager to show off to her classmates. The bell rang, and she joined her friends as they lined up to go inside. There was some pushing and shoving in the line, but Heather patiently waited her turn, holding fast to her bathing suit as she filed into the school and out of my view. She had not noticed me, which was just as well. I smiled to myself and went to the school conference. I was happy to learn at the meeting that what I had seen in the playground was generally true. Heather was truly part of the school community, bathing suit and all.

* * *

I first met Heather when she was four years old and had come for a
diagnostic assessment. When she marched into the office with her bathing suit firmly clutched in her hands, I asked whether she had just come
from the pool. Without pausing to answer, she rummaged around the
toy box and started to line up some tiny figurines, not an easy task with
one hand wrapped around a bathing suit. I turned to her mother, and
we got down to the work of finding out what her concerns were and
what might be done about them. I spent the next couple of sessions getting a history from Janice and playing with Heather, all as a way of collecting the information I needed to complete the assessment.

Separated from the children's father when they were very young,
Janice was raising Heather and her older brother alone while working as
a waitress at a local restaurant. Janice first became concerned about
Heather at around six months of age, when she noticed that her baby
did not seem to cry very much and was content to lie in the crib for
hours without being picked up. Compared to her brother, who had
been quite colicky as a baby, Heather seemed to be too placid and quiet.
Janice took Heather to the doctor when she turned one, because she
was not yet communicating her wants and needs, but he shrugged off
Janice's concerns. When Heather's speech did not improve, Janice persisted in telling the doctor that something was wrong, and eventually
she was referred to a pediatrician who decided that Heather had a
speech delay. That led to a referral for speech therapy at our hospital.
There, the speech therapist confirmed Janice's suspicions that more
than speech was wrong with Heather and that this extreme placidity
was a bit unusual, as were a number of other behaviors. The question of
ASD was raised, and Heather was referred to me at that point.

Although Heather was speaking when I saw her, most of her speech
consisted of phrases from TV and various children's videos. She always
carried around these silly bathing suits and would become very upset if
she couldn't find them when leaving for school or going out to her
grandparents' house. She restricted her diet to honey-coated cereal for
breakfast, lunch, and dinner. She refused to have her hair brushed and
was quite content to walk around with an enormous tussle of blonde
hair sticking up all over the place. She would line up little figurines in a
long row that stretched out across the room and down the hall and refused to play with her brother, who was just a year older. She cried every time her mother picked her up in her arms and was most content to
be left alone to stare at the figurines or to watch TV. She avoided eye

contact, rarely smiled, and showed little interest when her grandparents came to the house to visit.

Naturally, Heather's mother was very confused at first by her daughter's behavior. Why did she carry around the bathing suit? Why did she eat only honey-coated cereal? Why would she refuse to have her hair brushed? But above all, why did she not want to play with her mother? Why did she not seem interested in her mother at all, in fact? What was the source of the distance between them? This was the most difficult and painful question to pose. The answers that she feared might be true were the very ones she gave herself in the middle of the night: She worried that she was a bad mother, easily angered and frustrated. She had taken Heather away from her father at too young an age. She did not have enough money to buy Heather the toys she wanted. Perhaps Heather was enraged at her mother? The whole thing was obviously entirely her own fault.

In the face of uncertainty, we often fall back on "easy" or simple explanations; we personalize events and feel that they must be our fault. Janice's inability to understand her daughter, her behavior, and her eccentricities led to feelings of guilt, and that guilt put a strain on their relationship. Without understanding Heather, she could not get close to her. It was as if Heather was a shadowy figure in her mother's dreams. Instead of a feeling of closeness, guilt and recrimination rose up inside her and occupied her inner life. As a result, Janice lost her patience with Heather, she became irritated with her, she found it difficult to parent her, she could not tolerate her being so "different." Why couldn't she be like the other children at day care? All of Heather's difficulties were an accusation of her mother's failure as a parent.

Starting with our very first visit, Janice expressed this terrible sense of disappointment and loss. What Janice wanted most was what all parents want—a loving relationship with her daughter. What she got instead was a sense of exile in her own home. As long as Janice turned on the TV, got the right video, and put the honey-coated cereal in front of Heather, her daughter was happy. But there was little connection between them over and above these purely instrumental gestures. Heather didn't seem to need the personal closeness that her mother desired so much. In fact, Heather seemed to ignore Janice, to be almost indifferent to her mother's comings and goings, to view her mother as less important than her toys and TV. There was no sense that mother and daughter were together sharing an adventure, discovering the world.

When I finally completed the assessment, I remember the shock and disappointment that swept across her mother's face when I said, "I'm afraid Heather does have an autism spectrum disorder." I let the news sink in for a moment before asking Janice how she felt about that. "I was afraid you'd say that," she replied. "I was hoping for a different answer, though." There was an awkward pause as Janice rummaged through her purse for a tissue. Her next statement was delivered with determination to keep the tears out of her voice: "OK, now I want to know what I can do to help her."

In that simple declaration I recognized the process that begins with a flicker of recognition that a child is not developing as expected and then suddenly takes shape and crystallizes, becoming as hard as granite in the pit of one's stomach. In response, parents begin a desperate search for a sense of direction. When they hear the term "autism," a gaping hole opens up at their feet. The only way to fill it is to offer knowledge about the disorder, knowledge that leads to hope and a sense of mastery. Plank by plank, the hole gets covered up, and the first board to be laid is knowledge.

The information that parents want most is what treatment strategies are effective in building skills and in reducing autistic behaviors. While this is extremely important, at the same time it is essential that parents understand the disorder—the range of symptoms that impair all aspects of functioning and how this manifests itself in day-to-day life. In this way, the disorder begins to make sense; it is no longer so mysterious and impenetrable. The most important by-product of this type of knowledge (as opposed to concrete treatment strategies) is that a sense of connectedness can be reestablished between parent and child that washes away guilt and does away with that sense of exile.

So Janice and I started to talk about developing a treatment plan. Janice wanted to know what the problems were that should be addressed and what their relative priority was. What are the most important skills the child needs to learn in order to move on to the next stage of development? We agreed that Heather's restricted diet and her refusal to have her hair brushed were surely important problems, but these could wait until after we had worked on her ability to go to grade school, as she would be expected to do soon. But to be successful at school, she needed first to show more interest in social interaction. Unless she valued that, she would not be able to pay attention to the teacher rather than to objects of her own peculiar interest. She would not be able to learn more about the world and other people. And the best place to start in building a positive social relationship was to improve things between mother and daughter.

While we waited for extra help at school, we decided to put aside discussion of concrete treatment strategies for the moment and focused on understanding what made Heather think, act, and feel the way she did. It was a matter of entering Heather's mind and seeing the world as she did. This is a form of understanding that is harder to achieve than knowledge of concrete steps in a treatment plan. It is a more emotional, empathic, and intuitive form of understanding, but it still depends on what we know about ASD and how the process of impairments in social reciprocity and in perception derail development. With this understanding, parents can begin to develop a social relationship with their son or daughter, and this in turn leads to the slow resolution of grief and guilt that all parents experience once the diagnosis is given. Understanding of this sort leads to an acceptance of the predicament without resignation, a sense of hard-won repose.

Janice watched her daughter carefully and tried to see the world as Heather did. She imagined how certain textures must feel if their intensity were magnified tenfold. She stared at the patterns in the rug on her living room floor and was amazed at the intricate designs created by the play of light and shadow as the sun moved across the window pane. She started to carry around a shiny stone in her hands, almost like a talisman against anxiety (a bathing suit would surely be going too far, she assured me). Janice wondered what it was like to have a different sensory threshold. She tried to imagine having her hair brushed as if someone were pulling a set of nails through her scalp. She learned to hear how sounds that she used to be able to tolerate without difficulty, like vacuum cleaners or the alarm clock, could send Heather into a panic. She began to see how time spent alone, by oneself, was not so bad—it gave one time to pay attention to the patterns of things. Like Stephen's parents, she began to see the charm in her daughter's interests.

But beyond that, this understanding gave Janice a deeper appreciation for the communication signals that Heather did send. She became acutely aware that Heather did communicate, although it was atypical and not always received without distortion. With this dawning awareness, Janice began to realize that Heather's behavior was not so much that of a stranger or an alien who happened to live in the same apartment, but the behavior of just another child, whose world revolved around a different axis and who experienced the world according to a different set of parameters and fixed points. The confusion in her mind began to recede and with it the guilt and the sense of failure as a parent.

Once that was resolved, it was so much easier to develop a positive relationship with Heather. Slowly but surely, their time together was more interactive, meaningful, and productive. With that imaginative leap on Janice's part, they soon learned to play with each other: to line up the figurines together and play dress-up, first with the bathing suits but then with Grandma's old clothes. Janice learned to play at Heather's level, rather than expect her to play like other typical children and be disappointed in her failure to do so. She gave up trying to change Heather right away but concentrated on trying to understand her, to be sensitive to the behaviors that signaled a communication. As a result, Heather became more affectionate and would communicate to a greater degree her happiness and joy in the world of perception but also her distress at social interactions that had gone awry. This was a long process and was soon supplemented with the concrete strategies that are available to build skills and reduce challenging behaviors, some of which are described in Chapter 10. These two forms of understanding must go hand in hand if family life is to be reestablished and if the child's development is to get back on track.

*   *   *

Heather is still not "normal," to be sure. She continues to carry a bathing suit draped across her arm. If the conversation with her friends does not involve Pokemon, she quickly loses interest and drifts away. But the frequency of interactions with other children and her interest in being with them has increased. She is paying attention to the teachers at school and learning to read, write, and do math. The frantic and recriminating phone calls asking Janice to take her home have ceased. If she continues to improve at this rate, her prospects for the future are bright indeed.

By understanding her inner world, Janice was able to communicate more effectively with Heather and build a better relationship with her daughter. She was able to find a path to lead Heather toward the world of other people. But the journey changed Janice as well. She came to see that Heather's world had its own attractions and that these could (and should) be valued by others. Her daughter was unique, and such uniqueness was a gift. Heather had many special skills and talents that needed to be nurtured, not eliminated. At first, Janice was concerned that Heather would not fit in, would be different from the other kids at school and so end up isolated and rejected by them. Now she was learning that Heather saw things in a way that was of value to everyone. The patterns in the rug *were* beautiful when the light shone through the window. The bark *was* lovely as one moved around the tree. The diagnosis was not a defeat, a punishment for being a failure as a parent, but a different developmental pathway to be followed. Janice could now accept Heather's behavior without being resigned to it.

Heather once lost a front tooth and wanted her mother to pour water into her mouth to help the new tooth grow! She had a wonderful appreciation for how things develop. Janice learned a new appreciation for her daughter's developmental differences—without that acute sense of loss and mourning—by imagining Heather's inner world. That was something her daughter could not do for her mother in return, by the very nature of the disorder. So it had been up to Janice. All living things (teeth and children included) need nurturance and sustenance. Her reward was nothing less than positive changes in Heather, in herself, and in their relationship.

The long journey taken by Janice from that initial sense of disquiet that something is wrong to a new perspective on the world is a journey taken, in one form or another, by all parents of children with ASD. This book describes some of these journeys and is meant to be read in the space between hearing that one's son or daughter has ASD and beginning a treatment program. It is a dark space, full of shadows and uncertainty. Like Bluebeard's castle, parents fear that danger and disappointment lurk behind every door. Each possibility for the future may look more grim than the last, and perhaps the greatest fear is that one's child has been snatched away, kidnapped by some mysterious biological process. Into this space, this book is meant to find a place. Hopefully, these pages will open a window to let air and light into that dark room.

The thread that ties these stories together is that the sense of exile from one's child that parents feel is the result of not understanding ASD and how it affects the experience of childhood. The gaping hole that opens up at one's feet when hearing the diagnosis and seeing one's child on the other side of that hole is something that all parents feel when they first learn about autism. The emotional distance comes from the impairments in social reciprocity and in social communication that are a key part of the disorder. From this basic fault line flow the other difficulties—the restricted and odd play, the difficulties in learning, and the challenging behaviors. And from this comes the distance between parent and child.

As adults, it is our job to traverse that distance by entering the inner world of the child with an ASD. We cannot expect them to enter our world first, because that is the fundamental nature of the disability. Once we cross over, a transformation is possible—a transformation of the child, of the parents, and of all those who come in contact with somebody like Heather.

I can never look at the bark on a tree or a bathing suit the same way as I did before I met Heather. She moves all who stop and take the time to say hello to her along the road to confronting, then challenging, then celebrating diversity.

Chapter 3

Justin
Listening to the Architecture of the World

I often notice Justin pacing back and forth in the hallway while he waits for his appointment. Through the window he flits in and out of view as he goes up and down the corridor. He's always listening to his portable radio, just like any teenage boy. But Justin is thirty years old, and he lumbers rather than walks, humming a tune from the radio under his breath. I've known him for almost twenty years. He was one of the first people with autism I met, and for that reason he will always hold a special place in my heart. I've learned a great deal from Justin, and if he has benefited from my interventions, it will have been a fair trade. He has been through a great deal, and his parents, Mark and Vera, have weathered many crises over the years.

The nice thing about Justin is that he is always smiling, though this does not mean that he's always happy. He is a charming mixture of incongruous characteristics. His mouth smiles, but his eyes are often melancholy. He speaks in a flat monotone voice about a number of worries that plague him. But he smiles even when he talks about these terrible fears. He is now slightly balding and putting on a bit of weight. Justin usually wears a heavy coat, even in summer, and always sports the inevitable earphones. Often I have to remind him to take them out so we can have a better conversation. He looks at me quizzically and then reluctantly complies.

Jason is very attentive to sound when he comes to visit. As he

walks through the outer office, he notices all the computers and immediately classifies the CPUs as to the number of megahertz: 500 (too
slow), 1.2 gigahertz (better), 2 gigahertz (OK, but still not the best).
Apparently, each has its own distinctive sound as it turns on, performs a
function, and then turns off. The higher the pitch, the better the sound.
Justin loves machines that make a whirring sound—videotape machines, washing machines (especially during the spin cycle), dryers,
and vacuum cleaners. He was able to tell his parents well before anybody else noticed that their outboard motor at the cottage was running
on only two cylinders and should be repaired. Justin has always wanted
to work in a laundry or a dry cleaning establishment. The sounds that
the washing and drying machines make are pure joy to him. Some years
ago he found work at such an establishment, but he became so absorbed
in the sounds that he could not pay attention to the demands of the job
and was eventually let go.

Justin has always loved sounds. Even when he was first assessed
some twenty-five years ago, his medical chart specifically mentions how
interested he was in auditory stimulation. If asked today, he'll confirm
that he's always found noise and sounds interesting—that they give him
a sense of general pleasure and enjoyment. Sounds make him feel at
home: "Some are securities for me," he says. He once explained to me
that the experience of listening made him feel relaxed and at ease, even
"high" at times. He recognizes that this absorption in sound is not a
normal inclination, but he doesn't pay any attention to his differences
from other people. He can play the piano reasonably well but not ex-
pertly. He has a fine singing voice that is surprisingly free of the unusual
intonation of his speech in routine conversation. He is a perfect mimic
and can imitate his old high school teacher to perfection, especially the
one time he tried to teach the class about how washing machines work.
He giggles delightedly when he tells me this story.

Justin is especially fascinated with thunderstorms. Every time there
is a thunderstorm he takes his tape machine outside and records the
sounds. Afterward he plays the tapes to amuse himself and to help him
fall asleep. He also likes to buy commercially produced weather tapes
and will add them to his collection of homemade tapes. Once, after he
bought a couple of tapes, he quickly noticed the same thunderstorm
was on both of them. He was not a little put out at the discovery. "How
dare they try to pull a fast one on me?" he said indignantly.

I once asked him why he recorded thunderstorms. "They all sound
the same, don't they?"

Justin looked at me as if I were the stupidest person on earth. "No," he said. "They all sound quite different." But he did not elaborate.

I asked him to bring some tapes to our next appointment, and we spent the hour listening to them. He was right; all storms do sound different. He pointed out the variation in the peals of thunder. There were differences in volume, of course, but I had never heard the wide range of pitch and rhythm. How amazing!

Justin has the capacity to hear things that I am incapable of hearing naturally. It is this attention to perceptual detail that is so remarkable. But in a more general sense, it's the pleasure that the intricacy of detail brings to people with ASD that is so extraordinary. Children with ASD tend to love sounds, even more than typical children enjoy music. It is pure acoustic sensation, the rhythm and pitch that attracts and holds their attention. The words are of little interest, and the emotions conveyed in the lyrics are quite irrelevant. Asking the child with autism the meaning of a song will evoke little response over and above a repetition of the lyrics. I remember one little boy with AS who enjoyed drumming so much that he spent hours in the garage imitating the sound of the rain falling on the roof by banging on a set of boxes of different sizes.

I love music too, and to that extent I am not immune, at least intellectually, to the concept of experiencing pleasure at hearing pure sounds. I can even enjoy listening to very modern atonal music for short periods of time. But the music must have a narrative of some sort. There has to be a *reference* to something outside the acoustic sensation; the music must evoke emotions, images, or ideas. Without these external referents, I get bored quickly. My attention span for pure acoustic perception is very limited. I can force myself to pay more attention, but the effort required is substantial, and I quickly become exhausted. In my experience, most parents of children with ASD are just as mystified by their child's fascination with perceptual detail and quickly become bored by paying attention to a single repetitive stimulus for long periods of time.

For Justin, listening is effortless, and he is never bored by sound. Thunder is a compelling experience, not a nuisance to be avoided. The Dutch novelist Cees Noteboom writes that "boredom is the physical sensation of chaos." In precisely that way—as a physical sensation—thunder is a deep and meaningful experience for Justin. It is the antithesis of chaos; it is structure, routine, and the perception of ordered meaning. As such, it provides Justin with genuine pleasure.

Justin gets bored by other things, to be sure. But these are often the things that so interest ordinary people: novels, TV drama (but not sitcoms or comedy like the Three Stooges, which he loves), stories of general interest, and history; in other words, events that involve people, their social relationships, and their emotions. *That* is boring for Justin, not the sound of rain and thunder. "How could anyone consider that boring?" he asks me innocently. I suspect there must be a neurology of boredom; there must be a place or, more precisely, a set of neural circuits, in the brain where boredom is experienced. The function of that set of brain circuits must be altered in some subtle way in people with ASD so that they never tire of pure repetition.

Justin sits across from me today as he has on and off for the last fifteen years. He twists his curly hair and blinks frequently. He has that fixed smile that never wavers even though we talk about both happy and sad things. No matter the subject, the smile remains very engaging.

Justin has a lot of anxieties today—about being too physically close to people, about harming people, about his bodily functions, his stomach, his weight, his appearance, whether he has body odor, and so on. Some years ago, he developed a true obsessive–compulsive disorder that centered around cleanliness. It is not uncommon for higher functioning adolescents and adults with ASD to develop this type of anxiety disorder. Justin experienced frequent and troubling intrusive thoughts that he was "dirty" and "smelly." He would take frequent baths and would wash his hands many times a day. These anxieties and worries were an added disability for Justin since they also made him extremely irritable. He was often difficult to live with and very unhappy. He would lash out at other people in the group home where he lived , ask the same questions of others over and over again, and pace around the building. We were able to deal with these symptoms with medication, but paradoxically his interest in sounds decreased as a result. "They don't turn my crank as much," he announced sadly to me one day. "I don't feel any life inside me anymore. I'm a dead battery." This occasionally happens when people with ASD go on medication, and it certainly was a problem for Justin. We tried to take him off the medication, but he could not hold a job or live semi-independently. It was a difficult trade-off. Eventually Justin decided to take the medication in spite of the way it made him feel about the beauty of sounds, but we were able to lower the dose somewhat so that he still retained some pleasure.

* * *

Justin's love of sensation is common among children with autism and other ASDs. It's part of a larger pattern of restricted interests and activities that represents one of the most important aspects of the diagnosis. In his original paper on autism, Leo Kanner (see Chapter 1) framed these behaviors as part of an "insistence on sameness." The children he described in that paper were fascinated with letters and numbers, spinning blocks, and singing songs. They engaged in many fixed patterns of behavior that produced sensations of various kinds, and they had considerable difficulty accepting even trivial changes in their environment or in their routine. Sixty years after the publication of Kanner's paper, we now believe that "insistence on sameness," rather than being a single construct, is probably made up of at least three separate components: restricted interests and preoccupations, rituals, and a resistance to small changes in one's environment and routine. To professionals and parents alike, it's not always easy to tell which behaviors represent which of those components. Is insistence on lining up little toys on the carpet in a certain order the child's way of pursuing a restricted interest in those toys, or is it a ritual? Is having to wear the same blue socks every school day a ritual or resistance to little changes in routine? If we focus only on the fact that all these behaviors make the child "different," the distinction probably seems insignificant, even irrelevant. But it's important to think of the three types of insistence-on-sameness behavior separately as each may have a different meaning for the child and require a slightly different intervention.

Restricted interests and preoccupations serve as replacements for more typical forms of play. All children with autism and most with AS lack the capacity for highly imaginative and creative play. They rarely make up stories or use toys to enact those stories. Typical children will put little people in and take them out of a toy bus as it travels from stop to stop, or they may play out an extended sequence of grooming, bathing, and feeding a favorite doll. Without the ability to play imaginatively, the child with autism or AS pursues a set of circumscribed interests that seems to replace imaginative play and becomes a preoccupation. The child engages in these activities frequently, in exactly the same manner. I have known children who would watch a single video hundreds of times or line up a train set in exactly the same fashion, day after day. It's not necessarily the object of the child's interest that seems odd—there is nothing unusual about a girl liking fluffy toys or a boy being fascinated by sports statistics. Rather, it's the intensity with which the child participates in the activity that is so different from the habits of typical children and that may appear odd to adults. The child may become absorbed in an activity for hours without interruption (much longer than typical children can play) and protest if taken away or prevented from getting involved in it in the first place. A child with autism or AS is likely to ignore a parent's requests to come for dinner or to get ready for school, not out of stubbornness, as may be the case with typical children, but out of an intense preoccupation with the interest at hand, almost as if the child were under the spell of a sensation.

These restricted interests and preoccupations are different from other insistence-on-sameness behaviors in at least one important way: The latter are often associated with some distress for the child. Children with autism and AS feel anxiety when their routine or their environment is changed, so they avoid such changes strenuously. Both resistance to change and rituals are compulsive in nature; the child seems to have to do what he does to keep the world as constant as possible. It's almost as if those with ASD feel nostalgia for a perfect world, and they try to re-create that experience over and over again.

Rituals are fixed sequences of behaviors that are repeated endlessly in exactly the same fashion, like closing all the doors in the basement for no apparent reason or touching the stove every time the child passes through the kitchen. These rituals serve no obvious purpose and may also be a way of dealing with anxiety. For Justin, one ritual involved taking the same route to school day after day. If the bus driver had to change his route for some reason, Justin became extremely upset and caused a disturbance on the bus. He resisted change elsewhere too, becoming very agitated if he was not allowed to sit at the same place at the kitchen table during meals.

Behavior like Justin's can obviously create problems, because in our unpredictable world we are expected to adapt to changing circumstances, to go with the flow of things when doing so serves the greater good. But Justin can't do that. Whether it's the bus driver or a supervising adult at his group home, one can imagine how the response to resistance to change will depend on understanding the meaning of the behavior. If the bus driver understood that a change in route causes Justin great discomfort, would he throw him off the bus or call the police when Justin makes a scene? If a mother knew that a child has to wear blue socks to feel secure in going off to school in the morning, would she tell him to stop making a big deal out of such a little thing and send him on his way, as one might with a typical child? These are examples of the way in which understanding the meaning or function of a behavior modifies our approach to dealing with it. A parent's job is made more difficult, unfortunately, by the fact that it's not always easy to trace behavior back to the compulsion to resist change. In fact, it's not always clear that the person is struggling with anxiety, as aggression can often be the presenting problem.

As to restricted interests, there is an almost infinite variety of topics or objects that catch a child's attention and may become a fascination, even a preoccupation. The common element is that the preoccupations all lack social–emotional content—stamps, but not the personality of the person depicted on the stamp; flags, but not the people who live in that country or its history; sports statistics, but not the dynamics of team play, and so on. The content of the preoccupation may also change with the child's development. In infancy, the interests are often highly perceptual and include visual stimuli such as the TV, spinning toys, flashing lights, letters or numbers, textures such as hair and silk gowns, or sounds such as songs, music, and the like. As the child matures, the topics may become more conceptual in some ways, but they remain concrete: action figures, robots, flags of the world, astronomy, bus time tables, medieval knights, subways, dates in history.

But some aspects of the preoccupation never change. The hobbies and interests are always pursued with unusual intensity and most often alone. Their primary purpose is not a means of facilitating social interaction. Typical children may develop unusual interests too, but these are often a way of meeting other children and making friends. Indeed, typical children are usually very sensitive to peer influences in their choice of play materials and interests (a fact that toy manufacturers are well aware of). For the most part, children with ASD do not care what other children think about their interests and pursue them with or without other people. If others join in, so much the better, but *only* if the activity becomes more fun that way. Watching a ball fly through the air may be more fun if Mom or Dad throws it back. Two people playing a computer game may be more fun than one.

The fact that cooperative play is usually motivated in this limited way does not mean, however, that a parent cannot exploit common interests between a child with ASD and another to help the child with ASD develop social skills and relationships. As described in Chapter 7, deep and meaningful social relationships may blossom when two people with ASD have similar interests.

Why some children love letters or numbers, why others like Justin

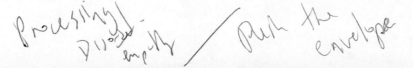

love sounds, and why still others become fascinated with esoteric subjects such as bones of the hand is an enigma. On occasion, another family member has a similar interest. I remember one boy who was obsessed with trains and insisted that his parents take him out for a drive every day to watch the 4:15 train pass over the bridge near his house. If they refused, he would become inconsolable. I asked his parents if they had any idea where this interest came from. They rather sheepishly informed me that the father was a steam engine enthusiast and had several model trains in the basement. The boy who was fascinated with bones in the hand and could recite the names of all the bones by the time he was four years old was the son of a chiropractor. Presumably he came across one of his father's books at a critical time in brain development and became hooked as a consequence. But this coincidence of interests is unusual, and for the most part, the reason a child has one interest and not another remains a mystery.

The mystery can be viewed as charming, as was Stephen's fascination with wasps to his parents (see Chapter 1), or it can cause great frustration. Some parents, naturally, have a hard time tolerating such eccentricities. After all, it can be exhausting to go to the extreme lengths that some parents and teachers have to go to in order to head off the difficult and aggressive behavior, particularly in young children, that often results when children are interrupted in the middle of their focused pursuits. But the reaction of parents and other adults to these interests is important. It may be very difficult to shrug off comments by well-meaning adults that point out how cute or how different their child is from other children—"He sure loves to line up trains all over your rec room floor. I wonder if he will grow up to be a train engineer?"—when you're trying to prevent such behaviors from occurring in the first place. But given the pleasure that these activities induce in children with ASD, such restriction will often only produce more difficult and disruptive behavior as a means of protest. As Heather's mother, Janice, found out, efforts to pull a child with ASD away from her peculiar interest to do schoolwork or chores or to play with the kids in the neighborhood can be futile. Chapter 2 describes how Janice and Heather's teacher found a way to capitalize on Heather's interests to increase her attention to the activities that developing children need to mature.

Some interests, admittedly, are dangerous. One little boy was so fascinated with the exhaust pipes of cars that when a car was idling on the street or in a parking lot he would bend down and watch the exhaust escape. Fortunately, it's more common for a child's intense interest to be a nuisance, especially because it is pursued with such intensity that it severely hampers family life. Parents cannot wait for hours while the child opens and closes the garage doors with the electric openers. I knew one couple who was, to say the least, annoyed when an enormous heating bill arrived in the mail, thanks to their son, who loved the sound of the furnace so much that he played with the setting on the thermostat. He made the furnace come on at regular and frequent intervals, even in the heat of summer, and each time it did, the sounds brought him great pleasure and excitement.

But as with Stephen, sometimes the interests can seem quite charming, and in those circumstances parents may take great pleasure in their child's preoccupations. I vividly remember little Chris, although I saw him only once since he lived far away. He was a lovely boy with short dark hair and big green eyes. The family lived out in the country by the banks of a small river. Along the river were tall aspen trees that could be seen from the backyard of the house. Chris became very excited whenever he watched the wind blow through the trees. The branches swayed, the leaves rustled and shimmered in the sunlight. Chris would stand there in his backyard, flap his arms, and make humming sounds. He loved to watch the trees move in the wind. Then he and his mother would hold hands and dance, because, as Chris said, "the trees are dancing."

Whether or not these eccentric interests and preoccupations should be eliminated is a common question and one without a definite answer. To eliminate them entirely may not be possible or even desirable as they represent true play activities, and play is essential to the development of communication and social skills, especially if the play can be extended to include other children. Sometimes, however, these interests and preoccupations are experienced as intrusive and troublesome by the child, almost like the obsessions seen in obsessive–compulsive disorder (OCD). When that occurs, treatment with medication is certainly indicated. There is good evidence that the selective serotonin reuptake inhibitors (SSRIs) are effective for the rituals and obsessions in OCD and more generally for symptoms of anxiety in children with autism and AS.

When the interest is troublesome or intrusive, it is important to limit the pursuit of that interest to a time and place that does not interfere too much with the family or other people. Often the activity can be limited to the child's bedroom or else pursued away from people outside the family. This can be done by setting aside a certain time each day when the child is allowed to pursue his interests without interference from others. It's also helpful to try to broaden the interests to be more developmentally appropriate or to include other people. Children initially fascinated with computers can learn graphics or programming. They can play computer games with their siblings or with other children with ASD. These modifications can be accomplished using gentle persuasion, rewards of some kind, or even medication. The child who was preoccupied with car exhaust systems had to be supervised closely when out in the community and prevented from going to parking lots or playing in the streets. Instead, he was encouraged to draw exhaust pipes and to plaster his walls with his drawings. Eventually these strategies led to a decrease in his interests in the real thing, and he turned his attention to antique cars in general.

These interests and preoccupations may be on a continuum with the amazing skills shown by people known as savants. Attention to perceptual detail can be linked to remarkable memory abilities or the capacity to develop complex algorithms to solve computational problems, like knowing what day of the week someone's birthday will fall on far into the future. Most savants have autism, but some do not. Savants tend to be quite impaired intellectually, and so the ability to perform complex cognitive tasks that are beyond the capacity of most of us is all the more remarkable. True savants are, in fact, quite rare but have caught the public imagination for years. In the last century, Dr. Alfred Tredgold wrote of the Genius of Earlswood who could draw meticulous pictures of naval ships and insisted that he was an admiral, even though he lived in an asylum and had never been to sea. He was apparently quite a celebrity in Victorian England. There are lovely pictures of him in a naval uniform standing in front of one of the model schooners he had built. Other well-known savants in our own time have demonstrated astonishing artistic ability. Stephen Wiltshire is a person with autism in England who makes beautiful drawings of buildings, streetscapes, and cars. He has published several books, has sold many drawings, and more recently has attended art school, where his talent continues to develop even though on conventional measures of intelligence and language he is quite delayed. But he is able to use his attention to visual detail as a means of recapturing moments of perception as they happen in everyday life. Hikari Oe is the son of Kenzaburo Oe, who won the Nobel prize for literature in 1994. Hikari was born with a malformation of the brain but survived after a long and difficult operation. In addition to seizures and visual problems, he has autism and a prodigious memory for sounds and music. He was always fascinated with music, even as a baby, and as a young toddler he listened to his parents' classical records for hours. The story of his growth and development has been a major focus of his father's writings, a way of giving his child a voice. Today Hikari composes lovely music that is baroque-like, formal, and classical. The melodies are quite delicate and pristine, usually consisting of either solo piano or piano and flute. They are light and airy, without dark and brooding passages. His records have sold extremely well in Japan and around the world. Like Stephen Wiltshire's paintings, his extraordinary perceptual memory and attention to acoustic detail have allowed his musical talents to blossom even as the capacity for social relationships and language remain limited. These savants illustrate in quite dramatic fashion that the flip side of a disability can, on occasion, release a skill or a gift that is beyond what most of us can accomplish.

But to be amazed at the ability to calculate birthdays in the year 2050, to make meticulous drawings, or to divide astronomical numbers in one's head misses the point. What is so fascinating is the more common experience of pleasure that perceptual detail arouses in children and adults with autism and AS. Justin's acute perception of acoustic detail and Chris's attention to visual stimuli aroused by the trees dancing in the wind are intensely pleasurable—they are experienced as true play. Without a fully developed capacity for imagination, people with ASD turn to the concrete world of perception and explore it in all its variety and in its sameness. The pleasure that it brings is no different from the pleasure experienced by typical children as they play with toys and dolls. Even the play of typical children has to be limited and fit into the daily course of life's events.

It is the ability to see, hear, and play with the intimate architecture of the world that is truly amazing. The rest of us can see this architecture too if we make a conscious decision to look. But we are rarely drawn to it as a natural affinity. We have to work at it. We have to turn away from language and from social relationships to see it. People with autism gravitate to it effortlessly.

* * *

What is going on in the brain that gives rise to these repetitive, stereotypic interests and activities? What neurological mechanisms are responsible? Several theories have been proposed, each with both merits and limitations. One is that people with ASD lack an understanding of other people's minds; they have a real difficulty understanding the beliefs, motivations, and emotions of other people. As a result, they might find the social world frightening and bewildering, as Sharon, an adult with some characteristics resembling AS, describes eloquently in Chapter 5. Social interactions are either meaningless or else unclear and ambiguous to children with ASD, which may lead to confusion and stress. This may be particularly true for children with AS or milder autism, because they are likely to be integrated into the social world, where they are constantly faced with their inability to understand communication and social discourse.

According to this theory, people with autism turn to the perceptual and concrete as a refuge, a place where predictability is possible, where meaning does not depend on social context. In this explanation, the love of perceptual detail is *secondary* to loneliness and to the loss of the social world as a place of meaning. As a result, people with autism are given little choice but to develop an intense interest in perceptual detail. But this does not explain the genuine pleasure experienced by people with autism and AS when they engage in repetitive and stereotyped interests.

We might also expect to see a nostalgia for the social world, a deep and profound longing for social relationships among people with autism, and this is rarely the case. People with AS in particular (and, I believe, even those with more severe autism) do want to be involved with other people and certainly want to develop meaningful relationships, but loneliness is not the terrible emotion for them as it is for typical adolescents. It does not rule their lives as it might for many other young people.

Another theory proposes that people with autism have high levels of anxiety and arousal; they are irritable, sleep poorly, are overactive, and, like Justin, experience considerable anxiety as a natural consequence of their disorder. Their repetitive behaviors might act as a coping mechanism designed to soothe their anxiety and dampen their arousal. We know it's common for those with ASD to have unusual fears—of certain sounds, rain, elevators—and to feel a lot of anxiety about impending changes in routine or the environment. And we can see examples of stereotypic behavior being used to soothe anxiety and lower arousal levels every day when we see mothers rocking fussy babies. So it makes sense that people with autism might be using their repetitive behaviors and rituals to cope with their anxiety and calm themselves down. Likewise, we see adults with Alzheimer's disease use "insistence on sameness" as a coping mechanism for the anxiety that accompanies their dementia. But, while it's true that some people with autism and AS are anxious in social situations, many people with true anxiety disorders do not show the preference for repetitive stereotypic interests and activities that people with autism show. Moreover, children with autism and AS will engage in repetitive activities even when they are not feeling stress. On balance, therefore, it seems that these first two theories are not comprehensive enough to be helpful in explaining the origins of repetitive behaviors.

A third hypothesis is that these behaviors actually represent a type of OCD. It's true that people with OCD perform many rituals and engage in repetitive activities as well. OCD is an anxiety disorder, and there are many similarities between ASD and OCD, but these are more apparent than real. People often say that a child with autism is "obsessed" with spinning wheels. This is not precisely true. A true obsession is experienced as uncomfortable, recognized as nonsensical by the person enacting the behavior. Rituals in OCD are engaged in as a way of avoiding the obsessive thought, and, as a result, that ritual is also experienced as distressing. But most repetitive activities are experienced as *pleasurable* by children with autism and AS. It is fun, not something to be avoided. Indeed, many parents wish their child would avoid some of these activities. This is quite different from the emotion experienced by people with true OCD. Some people with ASD do develop true OCD over and above the ASD. But that may be quite a different phenomenon and often does not occur before adolescence.

Two other theories are perhaps more plausible and help to explain why children with autism and AS have such difficulty in imaginative play. Uta Frith and Francesca Happe note that people with autism have great difficulty in integrating perceptual information from a variety of sources but are better than ordinary people in seeing details. We see figures against a background and integrate information from both to generate meaning. In contrast, people with autism and AS pay more attention to the figure and ignore the background. The Embedded Figures Test clearly illustrates this ability. The person taking the test looks at pictures composed of many dots. Those who don't have ASD tend to realize that some of the dots make up a recognizable figure only upon looking very closely. Much more quickly than the rest of us, people with autism see those figures embedded in what, at first, looks like a meaningless tangle of dots. Frith and Happe interpret this ability as a preference for local information processing over global processing. This means people with autism cannot see the forest for the trees, but they see the trees in exquisite detail! This weak central coherence (as they call it) leads to an inability to extract meaning from the context of a situation. So people with autism and AS are stuck repeating the same stereotyped responses to the environment because they cannot integrate information from other sources to modify their behavior. They cannot use their knowledge of the forest to find a path through the trees. Imaginative play requires the ability to think of *this* plastic object as a doll and in turn to pretend that it is a real baby. The child has to go beyond the thing in front of her and imitate a repertoire of behaviors illustrated by a parent. That imitation integrates information from another time and place with the object in front of the child's eyes. Without that ability to imitate and integrate, the child is stuck with the thing itself, and the pleasure associated with play becomes attached to it.

The other popular theory proposed to explain repetitive stereotyped behaviors and interests is that people with autism suffer executive function deficits. Executive function is a general term referring to the voluntary control, monitoring, and execution of behaviors and actions. It allows the person to disengage from the immediate focus of attention in order to pursue a goal, taking into account all available information. In some sense, executive function represents the supervisory aspect of cognition. The ability to monitor one's attention to attain a goal resides in the frontal lobes of the brain. It is a complicated cognitive skill and is composed of many constituent parts.

One important part is the ability to *shift attention* voluntarily and effortlessly from one setting or stimulus to another. My colleague Susan Bryson has pointed out that people with autism have extraordinary difficulties in shifting attention from one thing that catches their interest to another stimulus, even if that stimulus is also of interest. This difficulty is apparent at a very young age and is often remarked on when parents say their child spends a lot of time staring at the mobile in the crib or at the TV. It may also explain why children with autism spend so much time in front of the computer or playing with the same objects over and over: Their attention gets "stuck" in the moment, becomes locked into a particular stimulus, and the ability to easily shift attention to something else is not available to them. This difficulty in disengaging attention (particularly visual attention) could lead to the child doing the same thing over and over again and becoming fascinated with perceptual detail. A child who cannot shift attention will tend to repeat behaviors and activities without variation.

Another important part of executive function is the ability *to gener-ate* a novel response spontaneously. To perform any new action, such as walking through the kitchen, we need to inhibit previously learned responses and generate a novel response to environmental stimuli and situations. In other words, we need to be able to take into account everything that is going on and relevant right now to decide how to behave as we walk through the kitchen. If on one occasion a child touched the stove on his way through the kitchen, deficits in executive function would make it difficult to inhibit that touching behavior each time the child walked through the kitchen. Perhaps a child with autism is unable to stop touching the stove because he cannot generate a novel response. That stimulus (the stove) always elicits the same response (touching). There is a subtle difference between inhibiting a previous behavior and generating a new one. In either case, however, spontaneity would be impaired, the ability to adapt to changing circumstances, to apply something learned in one setting to another context. As a result, the same set of behaviors would be seen over and over, and the ability to be creative and flexible in different situations would be lost.

We can see this vividly when we teach social skills to children with autism by helping them to learn certain rules (see Chapter 5). The child can memorize these rules and can then demonstrate appropriate application of these social skills in the laboratory. But the same child will not necessarily be able to use those skills consistently in everyday interaction in the schoolyard. It is almost as if she cannot incorporate what she has learned into real-time social situations. Perhaps that is why the social mannerisms of people with autism often seem so formal and pedantic. They look like they are acting, like they are applying memorized rules; the spontaneity of social chitchat is absent. There must be a neurobiology of spontaneity just like there is a neurobiology of boredom. Perhaps the circuits in the brain overlap.

The central coherence and executive function hypotheses can explain the fact that the behaviors occur frequently and in the same way, but the essential element missing in all these hypotheses is why engaging in the activity is so pleasurable. It is also hard to explain fully the social and communication difficulties experienced by people with ASD on the basis of weak central coherence or executive function. This is more easily explained by the idea that people with autism, and to some extent with AS, lack a theory of mind, discussed in depth in Chapter 5. The pleasure felt by Justin and Chris when engaging in their repetitive behaviors is palpable. Listening to thunder and watching the trees is fun, even if they do it over and over. Of that there is no doubt. Why should it give them so much pleasure? These fascinations and circumscribed interests are almost like an addiction, but an addiction to perception, to detail, to pattern and rhythm. In some sense, form, line, color, repetition, and movement are addictive for the person with autism and AS, but not addictive in the same way that other people become addicted to alcohol or certain drugs. That is the key mystery that resists explanation and, I suspect, will do so until we have a better understanding of the brain systems involved and the connection between the frontal lobes and the reward center of the brain.

*   *   *

I remember having a free afternoon in San Francisco some years ago and deciding to visit the art gallery. There was an exhibition featuring Robert Ryman, an artist who paints in the minimalist tradition. I had never heard of him, but with nothing better to do, I ventured inside. I was soon completely dismayed. The entire show consisted of hundreds of white paintings: big white paintings, small white paintings, nothing but white paint. This is ridiculous, I thought. This guy is pulling my leg. White paintings indeed! Modern art at its worst. Anybody could do this.

I soon noticed, though, that each painting was in fact subtly different. The size of the paintings ranged from quite large to quite small, but the brushwork also varied from painting to painting. Sometimes a large brush was used, sometimes a small one. Sometimes you could see the canvas showing through; at other times the entire surface was covered. Sometimes there were fasteners, or bits of white tape adhering to the picture; at other times the paintings seemed to hang in the air by themselves. Sometimes the paint was thickly laid on, sometimes only very thinly. In fact, once I paid attention to these details, the paintings displayed an almost infinite variety of aspects. It soon became fun to see all the ways the painter could vary the same details and what effect he could achieve in doing so. After a while I became amazed at the extraordinary richness of the paintings and stood in wonder before his achievement! What a paradox, hundreds of white paintings, each one very different. Obviously this artist was never bored with painting white. It was the physicality of the paint he was interested in, its thickness, the brush strokes, the texture, the size of the canvas, and so on. There was no figure and ground as there is with most paintings, no near and far, no shading and shadow. Just white paint, simple but applied with care and considerable thought. There were no obvious references to outside influences, no narrative. There was no grand expressive artistic gesture, no inflection of affect. He had painted literalness itself. Through simple repetition and a careful process of elimination, he brought to the spectator an acute sense of the physical substrate of the world, a world beneath the layers of language and metaphor. He had managed to see infinite variety in something so simple as the color white.

Viewing these paintings, I could see the potential variation inherent within sameness. I could see how one could be perpetually interested in visual detail and not be bored. This was a world of pure sensation, no more profound meaning than the diversity of the simplest things. For a brief moment, I suppose I had come to see the world in the same way as a person with ASD. The pleasure I experienced at seeing these white paintings must be analogous to the pleasure experienced by Justin listening to thunder and by Chris watching the trees sway in the wind. This artist had access to a level of perception that is commonplace among people with autism and AS. I know that Ryman is not autistic. On the contrary, he appears as typical as the rest of us. And I know that most people with autism are not artists. But Ryman has discovered, if not by design then by serendipity, the kind of world people with autism and AS live in. He has opened a door for us and allowed us at least to look in.

The crucial difference is that the artist can go back and forth between the world of perception and the social world. He has a choice. People with autism have no such choice; they are locked in that world. A life without metaphors is not without cost. People with autism and AS cannot reflect on their experience; language gives us distance from the perceptual and the freedom that comes with it. Metaphors free us up from the literal. Language even gives us the means to control the world, sometimes at our peril. The ability to see the perceptual world is inherent in us all, not just in Justin and Chris. This perceptual life has been released and probably magnified by the neuropathology of autism. In us, this ability is under constraints, chained to language and metaphor and social convention. But we can see it on occasion and so appreciate the mysterious ways in which human development can go awry.

Chapter 4

Zachary
An Obsession with Death

Not all obsessions have the potential to develop into passionate and intense interests that enrich perception. Some are terrifying in their implications. At age nine, Zachary was obsessed with death. He constantly asked his mother, Angela, "What happens when Grandma dies? Who will replace her?" He then systematically went over all the members of his family, asking the same question: "What happens when Uncle Jim dies? Who will replace him? What about cousin Sally?" Almost his entire conversational repertoire consisted of asking these questions. He could talk of little else. Reassurance had little or no effect, and choosing not to respond only made Zachary more determined and insistent. Naturally, his mother was very upset, worried about what this meant and frustrated by having to travel up and down her family tree over and over again. Zachary's insistence on asking the same questions led to all sorts of other problems. He could not leave her alone in the small townhouse where they lived or give her any peace while she was making dinner or trying to help him with his homework. He would even wake her up very early in the morning and go through his list of family members. If she did not answer in exactly the same way, Zachary would become even more upset. It was clear that he did not enjoy asking these questions, as he looked tired and worried. But it was as if he could not stop himself. He must have asked the same set of questions hundreds of times in the last few months.

Angela was raising Zachary alone while working as a clerk in a bargain store. Her dream was to become an actress, but these aspirations had to contend with her son's disability. With this added stress, there was little likelihood of finding the time to pursue another career.

Why does a nine-year-old boy become obsessed with death? How can this be understood in a child with ASD? What is a parent to do? Angela asked to see one of our therapists to discuss these questions and to find a possible solution to the problems it was causing for both her and Zachary. While they were having a conversation in the living room, a small, rather plaintive voice called out from the kitchen, "What about ol' Blue Eyes, then?"

Angela and the therapist looked at each other in despair. Frank Sinatra had just died the week before. Zachary was now extending his range of concerns beyond the immediate family. This was not a good sign and was another indication that Angela's attempts to deal with the problem on her own were having little effect.

Why Ol' Blue Eyes? Apparently Frank Sinatra was his grandmother's favorite singer. She had recently developed an ulcer. Perhaps Zachary was worried about the effect his death might have on her health—or so Angela surmised. Zachary could not articulate to his mother or to the therapist why he was worried about Frank Sinatra in particular.

I had seen Zachary some three years earlier for an initial assessment. In the interim, our therapists had worked with him and with his mother to address concerns about behavior in school and social skills with peers. But this time I wanted to see him as well. This sounded more like a profound problem with anxiety than a difficulty in getting along with friends and doing well at school.

It was nice to see Zachary after such a long time. He arrived one warm spring day after school. He had very short-cropped blonde hair, with little tufts sticking out haphazardly. He had grown quite a bit since I had last seen him. The most striking thing about his appearance was the way his legs and arms stuck out from his body. His tight T-shirt and shorts accentuated this gangly appearance, and he moved his limbs in a rapid, staccato manner. He carried several small toys with him— Volkswagens in green, red, yellow, and blue. When he came into the office, Zachary immediately went to the toy box and picked out a white police car. He did not actually play with it but rather held the car in his hands along with all the other small toys.

As if on cue, Zachary began to ask his mother the familiar questions: "What happens when Grandma dies? Who will replace her? What about Uncle Jim?" Angela answered him dutifully. I was amazed at her patience, but I could also see the fatigue in her eyes as she replied to the same set of questions she had answered hundreds of times before. Angela was powerless to withstand the relentless insistence of his questioning. She had tried several maneuvers to get him to stop—ignoring him, giving him a time limit ("You can ask me questions for five minutes and that's it"), imposing time-outs ("If you ask me one more time, you have to go to your room for a while")—all to no effect. There might be a momentary respite in his questioning, but it would be short-lived, and often he would return with even more insistence and anxiety than before, almost as if he were becoming agitated by the stress of restraining himself.

Zachary then blurted out, to no one in particular, "Denver on *The Dukes of Hazzard* died. He died of lung cancer. I'm going to watch the memorial on TV." *The Dukes of Hazzard* TV show was also one of his preoccupations, as there were several car chases in each episode. It turned out that the main vehicle is a white police car, just like the one Zachary held in his hands.

I asked Zachary what happens when you die. "You go in a casket, your body is buried and dug in the earth," he replied.

Most children his age believe that a loved one who dies goes to heaven and may return to visit—or some variation on this theme. I asked him if he believed in heaven.

"I don't believe in hell, and I don't talk about heaven," he replied. Very sensible, I thought.

"I don't think you come back," he went on. "Frank Sinatra was eighty-three years old when he died. He sang 'My Way.' " The conversation veered off in all directions, much like a car out of control.

I was astonished that Zachary had such a sophisticated understanding of death, one that contrasted so sharply with his interest in small toys. Most children with ASD have much more difficulty with abstract concepts like heaven and hell. But then again, I wondered if I was missing something important. Perhaps his understanding was not so sophisticated after all. Perhaps Zachary was simply repeating something he had heard others say at funerals or in conversation. In fact, his mother told me that in the previous year Zachary lost one great-aunt to cancer after a twelve-year illness and another great-aunt died at the age of ninety-two. Since then, there had been much discussion among extended family members about death, and it was soon after these events that his grandmother developed an ulcer. She was not seriously ill, but she was a worry to Zachary's mother, who relied on her a great deal to help out around the house and to look after her son.

"I call her Alice," Zachary piped up.

"Do you?" I asked, adding, rather stupidly, "Is that her name?"

"No," his mother interjected. "Her name isn't Alice at all. That's the name of the housekeeper from *The Brady Bunch*, another one of his favorite shows." I was trying very hard to keep this straight.

"At the same time his grandmother was ill," Angela continued, "the movie *Titanic* came out." He was not allowed to see it, but this has always been another favorite topic of Zachary's. He has read everything he can about the sinking of the great ship.

"It hit an iceberg," Zachary said, and made the sound of the ship's hull crashing into something. Zachary cannot listen to the movie's popular theme song without crying, his mother added. Then he became worried about all the main characters in his favorite TV shows dying. He scoured the newspapers, especially the entertainment section and the obituaries, and watched all the newscasts, looking for death notices. He constantly asked his mother who would replace so-and-so in the show if there was a death. Curiously, he never asked his mother if she would die and who would replace her.

I asked Zachary if he was afraid of dying. He has nightmares, he admitted. "I had a dream on a night about me having to go underground. What would happen to my spirit?" he asked his mother, but then answered himself with a rather grand theatrical gesture of the hands upwards: "My spirit goes up into the sky and goes in everyone's heart." This is an explanation his mother had given him to comfort him, but this was the first time she had heard of these nightmares.

"Does everyone get sick before they die? Not always. They die in their sleep." He continued to answer his own questions.

What began as an initial concern about the health of a family member had now grown to include all Zachary's interests and preoccupations. But his obsession with death extended only to those individuals of direct and immediate interest to him. He was not worried about the war in Serbia or the famines in Africa, and the death of Princess Diana had left him cold.

"What about Louie Brown?" he asked. "He died in 1845."

"What about Louie Brown? Who is he?" I asked.

"He was the man who invented Braille," his mother informed me. Braille was another one of Zachary's interests. He learned all about it in school many years ago, and it still carried an intense interest for him, presumably because of the visual patterns and the texture of the dots. The death of Ferdinand Porsche, who passed away that spring, was especially troublesome to Zachary. He was the man who invented the Volkswagen, his mother again took pains to inform me. She, at least, could see I was having trouble following all this.

Zachary would tell me of the deaths of various people, both famous and little known, and then his mother, serving as a kind of interpreter, supplied not a translation but a context for these statements. This was the only way I could follow what Zachary was saying to me.

I asked Zachary when these worries began to bother him.

"Things went crash in the last months of school," he told me as he peered over his car, using the analogy of a car accident to explain his understanding of events.

"What happened?" I asked.

"I was not listening, getting suspended. . . . Will he get mad?" Zachary anxiously asked his mother, again over the top of the car. It was clear that school had been another stress for him, as some children were now teasing and bullying Zachary. He was in a regular class without any special assistance. He was quite bright and always had relatively good marks, as long as he could pay attention. But it was clear to everyone in school that Zachary was different. When he was younger, his eccentricity was easily tolerated by his schoolmates, but, as time went on, he became a target of teasing and bullying. These forms of abuse can be terrible to witness and even more terrible to endure, especially if one has ASD and cannot make sense of what all the fuss is about. Zachary had little idea he was different and that he was perceived as unusual by others, especially those wanting to make an impression on their friends. But he was very aware of the teasing. He would come home from school upset, not wanting to go back in the morning. His lack of sophistication and social understanding made him an easy target. Being eccentric can be a heavy burden when you are nine years of age.

*   *   *

After the appointment, I had an opportunity to reflect on what I had learned. It was clear that Zachary's preoccupation with death was not a fascination; it was not an interest that gave him pleasure, as sounds did for Justin or wasps did for Stephen. Rather, the predominant mood was one of anxiety and distress. Zachary was clearly anxious about people dying, whether they were known to him personally or were part of his TV viewing and other interests. He had a worried look on his face; he paced around the house asking his mother questions over and over again; he was having trouble sleeping. He never spontaneously said he was worried about death—one might expect that from a more typical child—but nevertheless there was a feeling of anxiety throughout the entire interview that was evident in Zachary's actions. Children with ASD find it difficult to talk about their feelings; that is, after all, part of the disorder. Instead, anxiety is often signaled by certain behaviors: repetitive questioning, disturbances in sleep, pacing, and an increase in repetitive actions, such as finger flicking and rocking. It is also often accompanied by a more intense preoccupation with the child's usual interests, so that getting his attention to turn to something else (like coming for dinner or turning off the TV) can provoke aggression and temper tantrums.

Little is known about how common these anxiety symptoms are in ASD and how to treat them. One frequently encountered set of anxieties are specific phobias of an unusual content. As mentioned in Chapter 3, children with ASD can be terrified of bees or mosquitoes, rain or the fog—things that don't usually terrify typical children. For example, Stephen would become distraught if one of his balloons made an unusual sound when the air escaped. He was very afraid of the broken bits of balloon flying around. In contrast, typical children may become phobic about the dark, big dogs, or spiders, phobias that are more understandable. Some adolescents with ASD have more generalized worries about schoolwork, about being teased, about having girlfriends—but again, often with an unusual twist. For example, Justin would become anxious about being too close to people, about harming them, about his bodily functions and how these might influence others. Typical children are anxious instead about being separated from their parents, afraid that something bad might happen to them, or else they are very self-conscious, easily embarrassed about their appearance, their speaking habits, and their clothes. Children with ASD seldom have such worries and are rarely, if ever, embarrassed since this emotion requires a clear understanding of how others might perceive them. Another important difference is that typical children are able to articulate more clearly that they are worried. These and other emotions are more apparent from their facial expression and overall behavior than they might be with children with ASD.

However, the most common anxiety among children with ASD is about change. They will, as explained in the preceding chapter, try to avoid it as much as possible. Indeed, "resistance to change" was one of the core symptoms of autism described by Leo Kanner more than fifty years ago. Children with ASD want things in their personal environment to remain the same—always. So do most typical children, but the odd thing about resistance to change is that for children with ASD the anxiety is not about major changes in a child's life (like changing schools or moving to a new house) but rather about more trivial changes—painting the bedroom a different color, buying a new car, taking a different route to school, or hanging new curtains in the living room. Changes such as these can precipitate terrible anxiety and frantic attempts to make things return to the way they were before. The birth of a sibling or the death of the family pet often passes unnoticed or is endured with seeming poise and equanimity. But the changes that Zachary was concerned about were not necessarily trivial; he was concerned about his grandmother's death and about death in a more general sense. This was not resistance to trivial changes in his life. This was like an existential crisis, so unlike other children with ASD. I did not understand what was going on.

When a new symptom is difficult to understand, it's frequently best to go back to the child's developmental history to look for clues that the symptom was already present but in an attenuated or covert form at an earlier point in development. In this case, it made sense to see if the current anxiety was part of a more general tendency for anxiety in Zachary's developmental history. I decided to go over his early history again and to look for anxieties that were perhaps not apparent at first.

*   *   *

I reviewed everything I knew about Zachary to try to understand the origin of this anxiety about death. Of course I had known him only since he was age six, but I did have information about his earlier development. Zachary's mother first became concerned with him at around ten months of age, when he stopped making sounds. Eventually he developed speech and was talking in sentences by thirty months. After that his speech progressed appropriately, except that he had a funny way of talking; he sounded a lot like Ringo Starr. Even at that young an age, though, it was difficult to have a conversation with Zachary. It was true that his grammar and vocabulary were mostly age appropriate, but he only wanted to talk about Thomas the Tank Engine and bumblebees. He would not respond to other questions, preferring instead to remain silent. He was never interested in reading picture books with his mother but became fascinated with the phone book and loved to watch the credits at the end of TV shows. His favorite show was the Business Report because letters and numbers from the stock market were constantly being flashed across the screen.

Zachary was first seen by his family doctor because he was considered a difficult child and a bit of a loner in day care. However, as his language and motor skills were quite good, the family doctor did not feel there was a significant developmental problem requiring intervention. He was not assessed again until kindergarten, when his teacher noted that he was having difficulty paying attention in class; he seemed absorbed in letters and numbers and spoke little to her or to the other children.

As a six-year-old, he had a few friends but would play alongside them rather than together with them. If his friends were not interested in Thomas the Tank Engine or watching the Business Report, Zachary would play by himself. Adults found him entertaining as he could talk to them on a surprisingly sophisticated level. He was especially fond of asking adults what kind of car they drove. He would proudly bring out this information at family gatherings and amaze everybody there with his memory. Zachary liked to be the center of attention as long as people focused on his interests. He always had a very close relationship with his mother; he was quite affectionate with her and would spontaneously give her a hug and come for comfort if hurt. He would sit beside her while watching TV and nestle up to her. But Angela could not get him to look her directly in the eye during a conversation, and they could not play cars together in a truly reciprocal way. Zachary tended to tell her what to do and would resist her attempts to modify the play.

Unlike many children with ASD, specific phobias or resistance to change had not been a prominent feature of Zachary's early development. But there were slight hints of things to come. For example, he would become very upset (possibly anxious?) at the sound of the vacuum cleaner, the blender, or anything else that made a loud noise. But that was it. There was no evidence of difficulty in changing from summer clothes to winter clothes, no problem in changing brand names of food, no difficulty in having his bedroom furniture moved around.

Very little had changed in the last three years. Zachary's language skills continued to improve slowly; he learned more sophisticated rules of grammar, and his vocabulary expanded appropriately. But he retained the same interests and the same fearfulness about loud noises. He memorized the dates of all the fire drills at school and became very anxious as the time for a new drill approached. His agitation and restlessness would escalate, and he had more difficulty complying with his mother's requests. This was the only anxiety I could see that was present in his early history and that continued to be a problem. But there seemed little analogy between this fear and death. The origin of his current anxieties about death were still a mystery to me, but he did seem to have a propensity for anxiety, a temperament to react in an anxious way to stress. I had to seek further for answers. Perhaps thinking more deeply about the content of his anxieties would help me understand.

*   *   *

In going over the interview in my mind, I wondered if Zachary was really anxious about death. Was it really possible that he was upset about the death of his two great aunts? After all, he had hardly known them. That he would be upset about his grandmother's illness was more understandable since he was quite close to her. Yet he had depersonalized her in a sense by calling her "Alice."

After rereading my notes from the interview, though, I realized that his obsession with death was quite different from what I had expected. I had taken his anxiety literally, much as one would do with a typical child worried about death and separation. His concern was not really an existential anxiety about the nothingness that follows dying; neither was it a romantic preoccupation with the glorious death of a childhood hero. He did not seem overly concerned with his own death or with his mother's death. There was no grief, no sense of mourning, no anticipation of the sadness that follows a death. Neither was there an awareness of the implications of death. There was no confrontation with the impossibility of knowing what happens after, no terrible wager with God. Zachary had never heard of Pascal.

Listening carefully to his repetitive questions about family members and other people connected with his interests, it became clear that these were not necessarily people he was close to, but more like objects, small toys off an assembly line. The obsession was not so much with death itself—the absence, the grief, the process of mourning—but with change and replacement. Every person had a replacement; the anxiety involved not knowing who that replacement would be.

This was a death reduced to its simplest, most concrete meaning as it related to him personally. What looked sophisticated on the surface was in fact a literal, entirely egocentric, interpretation of death. The important part of Zachary's interrogation of his mother was not the "What will happen to Grandma or Uncle Jim or Ferdinand Porsche?" question but the "Who will replace them?" question. More than anything else, I realized, Zachary was in fact terrified of change, of disruption in the order and coherence of his world. This was, in fact, the classic symptom of resistance to change, but because Zachary was so high functioning in terms of his language abilities, it appeared as a much more sophisticated anxiety about death and loss. My mistake was that I had paid too much attention to the first part of the repetitive questioning and too little to the second part about change and replacement.

Zachary had taken an abstract concept like death and reduced it to its most concrete dimensions. Zachary's language abilities allowed him to talk in a metaphysical way, but his ASD focused that concern on the immediate, literal consequences of death and the changes that it brings about. I had initially assumed that what concerned Zachary about death would be the same as it might be for a typical child. But I was wrong. The anxiety about death had to be interpreted through the prism of ASD, the distortion that the disorder imposes on a child's experience of the world and the vicissitudes of change.

In spite of myself, I found the whole conversation with Zachary amusing. So did his mother. We both found it funny that a nine-year-old child would have such an adult preoccupation and would express it in such a literal way. It made me remember a humorous scene from the novel *Molloy* by Samuel Beckett. Molloy is crippled and lives alone with his mother (whom we never meet). He likes to go to the beach and suck stones. He gathers sixteen stones and decides to place four in each of his pants pockets and the pockets of his overcoat. All his pockets are now full. His main problem is what to do with each stone as he finishes sucking it. He doesn't want to suck the same stone twice before he has sucked all sixteen. He decides to put a stone in his left coat pocket after sucking it but soon realizes that all sixteen stones will end up in the same pocket, an unsatisfactory solution. His answer is to rotate the stones from pocket to pocket, replacing each stone from his coat pocket with one from his pants pocket. He goes on and on like this, trying to find a perfect solution to the problem of replacement. He cannot deviate from the ritual of sucking the sixteen stones in turn. But of course there is no perfect solution to this dilemma; that is the point. It's a very funny episode but profound at the same time. The problem of replacing stones, which is silly at first, takes on a more conceptual, slightly sinister, and grotesque meaning through the device of repetition. Molloy's speech is a monologue on the problem of replacement. By going through his litany of repetitive questioning, Zachary too was engaging in a monologue about replacement, grappling with the problem of change. Only instead of stones, we were talking about people.

The anxiety and fear about change experienced by Zachary is just as profound in its own way as the more conceptually sophisticated experience articulated by Beckett, who can appreciate the absurdity of trying to achieve exact replacement perhaps better than Zachary. But the point is that these are universal experiences, accessible to all. Both expressions come from the same impulse. Death can be funny. Zachary does not know this, though; he is too focused on the literal consequences. In many ways the resistance to change that is experienced by children with PDD is like the nostalgia for a perfect world that we all feel; nostalgia for the time before the fall, when everything was plentiful and at peace. That perfect world can be the innocence of our own childhood, when there was a structure to the world, an order—one knew where to find things. That time and place is now lost forever (did it ever really exist?). No doubt, nostalgia is just our own resistance to change dressed up to be more respectable.

*   *   *

Now that I felt I understood the content of his fear and the meaning of the obsession with death, the form it took also made sense. The repetitive questioning was a coping mechanism for Zachary, a mechanism not uncommonly used by highly verbal children with ASD. Typical children use other, probably more effective coping mechanisms. All children, at one time or another, experience the same worries as Zachary, but they can articulate them in some fashion. The very act of articulation and naming, the bringing of language to a complex problem, often serves to reduce the resistance to change.

We are able to modulate our anxiety level for ourselves using language. We tell ourselves, in thought, that the world is not ordered, it is not perfect, nostalgia can be boring after a while. Perhaps language gives us this ability to put in perspective what makes us anxious, to look into the future and to anticipate a new order, to imagine a new way of dealing with change. Of course, the anxiety may return momentarily, but we can for the most part deal with it, sometimes by telling ourselves lies.

Due to their language deficiencies, children with PDD cannot verbally express their anxiety in ways that enable parents to recognize it as such, or to identify the true source of the anxiety. Although Zachary had good knowledge of grammar and vocabulary, there were still lots of examples of his difficulties in the social use of language to navigate his way through the world. I had a lot of trouble understanding what Zachary was talking about during our interview. He would bring up all kinds of people and topics without supplying a shared context for the conversation, in a sense engaging us and not engaging us in this conversation. Although I had never heard of most of the people he referred to, he seemed to have little appreciation that I might need some contextual information. The distinction between monologue and conversation was a tenuous one for Zachary. He made no concessions to the listener. Perhaps there is a connection between this difficulty in the use of language to navigate the social world and its ability to modulate anxiety. It is possible that his language skills could not be harnessed by his executive function skills to help him be aware of a listener's needs in conversation or to think of other coping mechanisms, of imagining another way of dealing with change. He cannot tell himself that it is of no use to worry about death because it won't happen to me, at least not yet. He cannot tell himself these sorts of lies.

Instead, Zachary's way of dealing with anxiety was to ask the same questions over and over again. This was unsettling and very trying for his mother. But for Zachary to be momentarily reassured, he had to ask the same set of questions over and over again, and Angela had to answer them in exactly the same way. The questioning became a verbal ritual, a means of warding off change. It represented his refusal to accept disorder. He must have felt that he was superimposing a whole different type of order over this anxiety—that repeated questions and the ritual of asking them were in and of themselves a type of predictability that supplied what the inevitability of change and death took away.

I could see this most clearly during the interview. Zachary had his set of lines to speak, and his mother had her set of lines. She had to deliver them in precisely the same way. It was the repetition, the ritual of asking the same question, that was momentarily comforting to Zachary, not the answers. It felt like Zachary, his mother, and I were in a little play. Zachary was both playwright and director. When I entered the theater, I too had my lines to deliver and my questions to ask. I was both actor and audience (certainly not the director). The play was a ritualistic reenactment of the anxiety of death expressed through the problem of change and replacement.

The relationship between ritual and theater is an old one, dating back thousands of years. Experiencing this conversation with Zachary and his mother reminded me that many of the earliest tragedies were attempts by the Greeks to understand death and how continuity was possible in a world where people die with some regularity. The audience knew the plays very well. The emotional power of the play was not in seeing how it ended, but in seeing it again and again. Repetition and ritual were at the heart of the healing power of the theater—and of religion for that matter. Zachary was, in a real sense, a part of that tradition.

Seeing this analogy between the experience of children with ASD—their anxiety about resistance to change—and the theater gave me a better understanding of the role of the repetitive questioning and the meaning of ritual as ways of dealing with death—or, in this case, the problem of change and replacement. My guess was that his grandmother's illness had made Zachary aware of the potential for his world to fall apart, for structure and order to disappear. The terrible teasing at school only reinforced his sense of not belonging and his isolation. The repetition was Zachary's way of supplying the structure and order that death threatens. He was using language to deal with the anxiety, but because of his disability it took the form of repetitive questioning. This verbal ritual and the need for reassurance about replacement helped him to cope and reestablish order.

But the added misfortune was that Zachary could not leave the theater; he could not put down the script and think of something else. As well as language, we also use distraction to deal with anxiety and change. We find things to distract ourselves—music, a good book, a brisk walk, or a pleasant meal. Zachary does not have the gift of distracting himself. Instead, he returns again and again to the source of his anxiety. His nostalgia for a perfect world is insatiable. The ritual and repetition are momentarily comforting; asking questions assuages his fear of change for that instant, but then it returns again and again. For Zachary the healing power of this form of ritual is incomplete. He cannot let go of his anxiety.

The ability to focus intensively on certain topics is both a gift and a curse. As a gift, it allows children with ASD to develop an extraordinary knowledge about cars, Braille, bumblebees, thunderstorms. But when the topic provokes anxiety, the gift becomes a curse. Children and adolescents with ASD cannot leave the danger of change alone and must return again and again to the source of their fear.

Our denial in the face of loss of order is very helpful. The ability to not see, the choice that we will not look at this now, will instead focus on something else, is another coping mechanism that saves us from experiencing anxiety all the time. Such freedom to be distracted is simply not available to children with ASD. They do not have the option of "not seeing." But, then again, we are often denied the privilege of seeing what they see.

*   *   *

Little is known about how to treat resistance to change as an isolated symptom. We do know that most individuals with ASD benefit from routine and structure. Presumably this helps them cope with change and the transitions that are a part of daily life. A schedule posted on the wall at school or on the refrigerator at home that outlines each day's activities with pictures and words is a common tool that makes transitions and change more acceptable. For example, when Zachary was in kindergarten, it was difficult for him to go from one activity to another during the course of the day. Once we understood the nature of his diagnosis, we suggested that the teacher make a set of photographs of Zachary doing different activities that were part of the daily routine. These were then placed in a prominent spot and were shown to him when it was time to make a transition. This led to fewer difficulties in going from one activity to another. We attempted the same thing at home to help with the routine of coming for dinner and going to bed at night. Again he responded well to these simple interventions.

But Zachary's anxiety about change at this point in his life was more abstract, almost metaphysical. A schedule placed prominently on the refrigerator would not help him deal with the changes brought about by death. A more useful strategy for Zachary might be to provide him with a new distraction. His extraordinary ability to become absorbed in a topic could be a viable way of helping him to forget his anxieties. If he could not imagine a new order to things through language, he would need a new interest to get him off the topics of death and replacement. The problem was that Zachary could not distract himself; we needed to do it for him.

This new distraction would have to be something special to provide enough impetus to help him leave behind the anxiety about change. Once we shifted his attention, with luck it might fasten onto another interest and leave the anxiety about replacement behind. To maximize the chances that this would work, we needed to take his favorite current interest and provide him with a new and exciting opportunity to indulge himself fully.

I understood from his mother that they would be going on a summer holiday and visiting the Henry Ford Museum in Michigan. Zachary was very excited about this trip as it afforded him an opportunity to pursue one of his passions—cars. This was exactly what we needed: an opportunity to have Zachary pursue one of his interests in an appropriate way by visiting a museum. Like so many other holiday tourists, Zachary and his mom could spend a day or two gazing in wonder at the sights and at the cars, though I felt sure that Zachary would be the only child there worried about the problem of replacement in human affairs. I hoped this trip would serve as a necessary distraction to pry him loose from his morbid thoughts and that he would be less anxious about death when he returned. Granted, going off to museums is not always practical as a distraction, but, then again, a preoccupation with death is not the usual form of resistance to change.

*   *   *

Indeed, when I saw Zachary later that summer, he was much more at ease about death and the problem of replacement. He did not scour the newspaper for obituary notices anymore, and he had stopped asking his mother the endless questions about death and who would replace whom on TV. It seemed like the distraction of the Henry Ford Museum had done the trick. He slept better, he did not look as worried, he was able to play by himself better, and there was less pacing around the house. He now even thought that *Titanic* was a crummy movie— another thing we could agree on in addition to not thinking about heaven.

It would soon be time for Zachary to go back to school. I hoped that the bullying and teasing would cease and that he would be afforded some peace by his schoolmates, so he could attend school free of anxiety. There is no escaping the fear of death, but there was no reason Zachary should bear the taunts from his schoolmates as well. He belonged in that world and had as much right to the stability and order that was possible there as the next child. As he left the office that day, I could not help noticing that his bulging pockets were full of small toys. When it comes to being interested in toy cars or preoccupied by death, cars become a wise and attractive alternative.

Chapter 5

Sharon
Seeing Other Minds Darkly

*T*he mail comes to the office in the afternoon, and I usually search through it quickly, hoping for a letter or two among the notices and requests. Sometimes the mail I receive is sad and poignant. Parents will write about delays in getting a diagnosis for their child or ask for another assessment, unsatisfied with their first encounter. Other letters ask about treatment options and what services parents should choose among the bewildering array of possibilities open to them. Other letters tell stories of children who are in trouble, who are teased by their classmates or are in danger of losing their school placement. Sometimes I receive correspondence thanking me for some small deed like writing a letter of support or giving a talk that proved helpful. I keep all these notes tucked away in a special drawer.

Some letters, though, catch me completely unprepared. One letter was written by an adult who wondered if people ever recovered from autism or AS. Sharon's letter began: "I would like to make an appointment for an assessment. Obviously, I cannot really be autistic, or even have Asperger syndrome since I have a husband, a child, and a career. But since I first heard of autism I have thought of it as 'my problem,' and this conviction only deepens as I learn more, and as I fail to change myself despite my best efforts. While professional diagnosis might be a comfort, professional denigration would be painful, which is why I have avoided exposing myself to anyone qualified to deny my self-diagnosis.

The main reason for writing now is the hope of finding a support group of fellow adult recoverees. I would really like to find some company."

A curriculum vita was attached to the letter. I learned that the writer was an architect who designed museums, private homes, and gallery spaces. Could such an accomplished person have ASD? Most of the adults I have seen with AS were still quite impaired in their level of functioning and what they were able to accomplish. But as we learn more and more about AS, it seems possible that some people with the disorder can be quite successful in adult life (Temple Grandin, described later in this chapter, is a notable example). Could Sharon be such an example? If so, I might learn more about the inner life of a person with AS and might learn, as well, how such people cope with the inevitable challenges that the diagnosis might pose. Perhaps new strategies could be devised from that information which would allow high-functioning people with ASD to cope more successfully with their difficulties.

Sharon thought this self-diagnosis was an accurate reflection of her predicament because she experienced significant problems in understanding and negotiating social interactions. She thought of herself as eccentric, and other people told her they often found it hard to communicate with her. In her professional dealings, she realized, on more occasions than she cared to remember, she had made some dreadful social gaffe with a client, but this awareness came to her only in retrospect and upon reflection. She felt uneasy with people, awkward and clumsy. Such difficulties are characteristic of people with AS but can also occur in people without the diagnosis. It would be a mistake to think that all problems of this sort are the result of ASD. Some people are shy; some people have a hard time successfully navigating the social games we play. But to give that predicament a medical diagnosis or to call it a developmental disability would be to extend the concept of ASD to such a degree that it loses meaning.

What intrigued me about the possibility that Sharon had AS was not only the types of social difficulties she described but also that she was an architect. This obviously required a high degree of perceptual skill and a penchant for seeing visual nuance and detail. In the letter, she wrote that people who are good at social interactions are often quite blind to physical reality: "Organizations are filled with people who are socially adept, yet they seem to be as blind to the material world as those with autism are to social reality. In physical reality, the existence of things cannot be denied. They may be understood and manipulated cleverly, but they never go away."

This was a fascinating insight. I wondered if she thought in pictures, much like Temple Grandin. Temple is an adult with autism who received her PhD in animal husbandry and became quite famous for designing a special cattle chute. She has written several books about her experiences growing up and what it was like to have autism. These books have had quite a beneficial impact on the public's understanding of autism. I have met her and heard her talk about how she thinks, not in words, but in pictures. This talent, an intrinsic part of her autism, allowed her to develop a career that made use of her disability. To even call it a disability is, in her case, questionable. In some individuals, the distinction between a disability and a gift or a talent is hard to establish. Was it possible that the author of the letter was an accomplished architect precisely because she could visualize the material world to a remarkable degree? If so, I could learn a great deal about how people with AS understand, perhaps in pictorial terms, their dealings with others and what strategies they use to overcome these problems.

Though I don't usually see adults clinically, I knew it had taken an enormous amount of courage to write and then mail the letter. Sharon said the letter had stayed on her computer for months before she mailed it. If I determined that she had AS, she might find a support group, and her sense of isolation might lessen. If not, I might be able to direct her toward more appropriate treatment or to other sources of support. I gave her an appointment with the intention of taking a skeptical approach. I would assume she did not have AS and would look for other reasons for her social difficulties.

For example, she might be depressed, and that might lead to a negative way of perceiving her interactions with other people. Or she might have some form of anxiety disorder. Some people who are very anxious feel uncomfortable in group situations. They are constantly monitoring their social skills, which are never quite good enough in their eyes. Some people are a little rigid; they may lack facial expression and are sometimes criticized by those close to them for being unresponsive or aloof.

Differentiating high-functioning ASD from other conditions can be quite difficult, more difficult than if the child has a developmental delay. The most difficult situations occur among children who are quite bright but have an anxiety disorder and a specific developmental problem in language or visual–motor coordination. The combination of the anxiety and the specific developmental delay can lead to social isolation as a result of shyness and poor social skills. Because they have nobody to play with, they develop a restricted range of interests that, of necessity, are pursued in isolation. The best way to distinguish these conditions is to search for difficulties in social relationships with parents and other family members that appear very early (before four years of age). The diagnosis of ASD is on firmer ground when children do not share interests and emotions with or demonstrate empathy for their parents. If all other explanations failed, I would entertain the possibility that Sharon had some form of AS. Perhaps she had some of the symptoms of AS but was very adept at compensating for her difficulties.

Sharon could be an invaluable resource because she would be able to articulate what many people with ASD cannot express. If we could learn how she was able to compensate for her deficits, we might be able to teach the same techniques to children with ASD. That would be a valuable learning experience for me. If I could help her in return, so much the better.

*   *   *

Sharon arrived at the office well before her appointment time and was reading in the waiting room when I introduced myself. My first impression was that she was quite apprehensive, but she greeted me skillfully and with grace. She was tall, well dressed but wore no jewelry (I learned later that she also never wore clothes with patterns, as these were distracting and made her nervous). After we settled some preliminary details, I began to collect the information I needed. I learned that she was forty-one years old, was happily married to a teacher, and had a young son. Her son was doing well in school and had lots of friends. Obviously he did not have ASD. Sometimes parents of children with ASD have ASD-like traits themselves, such as lack of social interests, poor social skills, difficulties in initiating and sustaining a conversation, or unusual hobbies pursued with remarkable intensity and interest. Here the link is genetic (see Chapter 8), and if Sharon's son had ASD, the nature of Sharon's problem might have been more obvious. However, that would have been too easy!

I asked Sharon why she thought she might have had AS. She took a deep breath and then proceeded to tell her story. She had always thought of herself as having very poor social skills and as being quite

eccentric, even as a child. Sharon felt that, more and more, these difficulties were getting in the way of her job and her relationships with
close friends and potential clients. Architects have to meet prospective
clients, understand what they want, and express themselves confidently
and precisely. They have to anticipate what the client wants, almost before the client finishes a thought. They need to exhibit considerable
personal charm in meeting with clients during the design process.
Sharon said she needed lots of explanation to help her understand what
other people wanted in the makeup of a building. She needed to write it
down and go away and think about it. Often during a conversation, she
had to repeat to herself what another person might be saying and de-
duce his or her meaning in a logical fashion. She also had to monitor
what she wanted to say in return and to make sure that it was not inappropriate. She had little intuitive understanding of others and had to
regulate her interactions with a continuous stream of self-monitoring.
She was, however, brilliant at being able to translate into visual images
and then drawings what the clients desired but could not articulate by
themselves. It was this skill that made her so successful as an architect.

Sharon knew that other people did not have these difficulties in
making social interaction as fluid and as automatic as possible. One day
she read an article about autism in a newspaper and experienced a flash
of recognition. She went on to do more research, including reading the
firsthand accounts of people with autism written by Temple Grandin,
Gunilla Gerland, and Donna Williams. Reading these had been a revela-
tion for her. What she originally thought was a personal failing or a
fault in her character perhaps now had a name and held out the hope of
greater understanding and of support from others with similar experiences.

I asked her to give me some examples of how she had coped with
these difficulties. She told me that, years ago, she had learned to write
rules in her head to guide her behavior. In this way she could compensate for her lack of intuitive understanding. She usually did this in bed
at night after a particularly humiliating day at school or at the university. Each social disaster was meticulously analyzed and categorized. A
rule was written for each situation and either added to the list or else
subsumed under some other more general rule: Look at people when
you talk to them; put out your hand to shake theirs; smile if they smile
when making a joke. Although this approach was generally effective,
the number of rules soon began to increase out of control. There were
too many rules to cover all possible social situations. Experience was

simply too varied to be cataloged in this way. Besides, the rules did not always help to govern behavior in the actual encounter. Often, Sharon could not remember the rules fast enough in the hurly burly of social interchange to avoid making a blunder. It was only upon reflection that the disasters of the day made their full impact felt. The realization would come to her that if only she had followed a particular rule, all this could have been avoided. The filing system that governed her social behavior was just not efficient enough; sometimes it let her down.

Through much of her life Sharon felt she could not intuitively understand what other people really meant when they said something. She took everything people said literally, without necessarily understanding the context. Neither could she see immediately that her own behavior was socially clumsy. She would comment on somebody's gray hair without realizing that the person might be offended, or she might tell a joke that nobody found funny over and over again. She would misconstrue their facial expression as puzzlement, not as boredom. Too often there was little correspondence between what she said and what she meant: "I spoke, and different meanings rushed in and attached themselves to my words. I seemed to be in a kind of time lag. I felt no meaning when something happened; only later, the meaning hit. Then in memory, I would really see what happened. Out in the real world, I was in a fog. I was never there at the moment something happened. First something happened, then, hours later, I felt it."

As she told her story I listened very carefully, puzzled but intrigued. These comments were precisely the kinds of experiences I had heard adolescents and young adults with AS describe when they reflected on their own experiences. I had heard from others bits and pieces of what Sharon was describing but never in one individual and in such an articulate fashion. This was quite remarkable. I asked whether she had any friends. She had very few friends, but those were very close and long lasting. It was very difficult for her to navigate social banter with potential acquaintances. She stated that she very much enjoyed being with other people but often felt so nervous that this anxiety seemed to get in the way of her social skills. She did not often initiate social interactions because she recognized that her approach was clumsy and inappropriate. She found it difficult to sense other people's thoughts and feelings and often felt detached from what was happening around her. For example, when she went to a sad movie it took her a while to understand why everyone around her was crying. She described difficulties in understanding the emotions of her friends and her own emotions in response to theirs. She could not see into other people's minds. She could see their facial expressions, their eyes, their smiles, yes—but not their minds.

To make up for this difficulty, Sharon visualized her own emotions; for example, anger was a whirlpool that she placed in a steel box, on top of which she planted a tree. It was not that she did not *feel* emotion. On the contrary, she felt things deeply and experienced a whole range of emotions. It was putting those emotions into language quickly and efficiently that was so difficult. Just like Temple Grandin, if she thought of emotions in pictures, they were easier to understand.

Sharon paused and looked down at her hands. This was obviously very difficult for her. I put away my pen and looked out the window. I distinctly remember seeing a lilac tree on the hospital grounds at the end of its bloom. The petals were strewn on the lawn like painful memories. My skepticism was slowly dissolving and was replaced with a growing sense of wonder and admiration. Sharon seemed to be describing the real-life experience of not having a theory of other people's minds, of being "mindblind" as Simon Baron-Cohen, a psychologist at Cambridge who has done a lot of the research in this area, calls it.

The idea that people with any form of ASD are "mindblind" is one of the most persuasive theories proposed to explain the kinds of social difficulties that people with autism experience. They find it very difficult to accurately understand other people—their motivations, beliefs, aspirations, and emotions. It is a difficulty in intuitive understanding, an inability to put themselves in another person's shoes and see their world from a social perspective. Our understanding of the minds of other people occurs because we carry an implicit awareness that lies just beneath conscious experience. These concepts are available to us almost by intuition; it is like an automatic way of knowing. We don't have to think about what to say after someone says hello to us; we know without thinking. Neither are we taught these concepts in a formal way by our parents but seem preprogrammed to learn them, in much the same way as children learn to use language. Our behavior, and the behavior of others, is interpreted in terms of inferred mental states that involve motivation, desire, and emotion. For example, if my spouse's eyebrows are raised, I infer surprise. If the corners of your brother's mouth are turned down, you infer sadness. We intuitively use our own set of psychological concepts to understand which motives, desires, perceptions, and emotions that are part of the experiences of another person are coming into play in any given social situation.

For the most part, we do this quickly and effortlessly—automatically. Typical children and adolescents do have difficulty reading social cues as well; of that there is no doubt. The difference is that this occurs from time to time, not continuously, and mainly for situations that are ambiguous. The difficulties here stem from a lack of maturity; they are not intrinsic to the person. For people with ASD, these difficulties occur in situations that typical children and adolescents would find obvious. It does not occur just in ambiguous situations but constantly. Moreover, people with ASD are often not even aware they are having trouble understanding the rules of social interaction. Typical adolescents are often acutely aware of their misinterpretation when it is pointed out to them, though they may not admit it to any parent or adult in authority. The difference is that for typical adolescents, it is emotions, impulses, or inexperience that get in the way of understanding social cues, rather than a fundamental cognitive deficit, as it is for people with ASD.

Young children typically begin to develop a basic understanding of other people's mental states between nineteen and twenty-four months of age, when they acquire the ability to pretend that a specific object is something else: This banana is no longer a piece of fruit but a telephone. This capacity to elaborate and use symbols soon evolves into social play activities such as playing Mommy or Daddy with dolls or with a younger sibling. By age four or five years, children have a remarkable sense of psychological mechanisms and can interpret and predict behavior by attributing mental states to their friends, their siblings, their parents, and themselves.

What is not clear is the form these skills take at different ages and how they are acquired. Some psychologists believe that children acquire psychological concepts much as they learn the meaning of grammar and words; that is, these are preprogrammed cognitive skills, hard-wired in the brain, that unfold with development and experience. Similarly, having a theory of mind may be hard-wired in the brain, but a child needs experience for it to be fully realized (just like children need to be exposed to language to utilize their hard-wired skills). Others believe that a theory of mind arises in a child from an ability to project himself imaginatively into another situation. By this account, children understand not by having a *theory* of other people's minds but by *simulating* imaginatively what must be going on in somebody's else's mind. A child might think that her mother is sad by intuitively imagining how she might feel under the circumstances and given certain facial cues. That emotion is then *projected* onto her mother. Understanding other's hopes, desires, and motivations might work in a similar way.

Beginning in the 1980s, experiments were devised to test this theory of mind (TOM) ability in children with autism and ASD. In the classic experiment, a child with autism is presented with the following scenario either with two dolls or two people: Sally puts a marble into a basket she is carrying and puts it down to go out of the room. Ann takes the marble and places it into a box that she has. When Sally comes back into the room, the child is asked where she will look for the marble: in the basket or the box. A child with good TOM skills will say that Sally will look in the basket because she does not know that Ann has taken the marble and placed it in the box. The child with autism, on the other hand, will state that Sally will look in the box, because he or she will not understand that Sally still thinks the marble is in the basket where she left it. The child with autism cannot read Sally's mind. It soon became apparent that most children with ASD did in fact have a severe deficit in this area, regardless of the tests used to measure TOM. What was so interesting was that the difficulties in understanding were specific to social situations; they did not apply to inferring simple visual perspectives that were not observable to the viewer. Children with autism could describe what lay behind a mountain or on the other side of a cube. They could describe what somebody else *saw* but not what the person *felt or believed*. This difficulty in perspective was also more than an understanding of emotions; it extended to motivations and desires and to all the internal mental states of other people. Both children and adults with ASD seemed unable to make a spontaneous, intuitive inference about the mind of another person and to have a limited ability to understand their own psychological makeup.

But it also became apparent that children with other types of developmental problems, like Down syndrome, had difficulties with TOM too, though usually their problems were much milder. There was also some concern that the tests used to measure TOM in fact captured a more primary problem in understanding the words we use to describe these concepts, not the concepts themselves. It may be that the children had trouble understanding the story or the meaning of what happened, not necessarily the mind of the dolls. After all, we have known for a long time that children with autism have considerable difficulties in comprehension and expression of language. But more recent work by Baron-Cohen has shown that even if the test is based on photographs of eyes and so does not require an understanding of verbal concepts, adults with ASD have trouble inferring accurate mental states from these pictures. In this version of the test, a person is confronted with a photograph of the eyes of another person and asked to identify the emotion or motivation experienced by that person. Even the brightest people with ASD have difficulty with this test.

The poor communication skills demonstrated by people with ASD can also be explained on the basis of a poor TOM. After all, to build a conversation with someone we have to understand what the other person is expecting in the way of background and context. We have to give the listener what he is expecting in the conversation. During the appointment it was apparent to me that Sharon had no difficulty in using language to communicate her experiences, but I asked her what it was like having a conversation with her husband, her friends, and her clients. She told me she saw herself as engaged in monologues with other people, not conversations. The conversation did not build through mutual discourse. She felt that she talked *at* people, not *with* them. To hear what other people were saying she had to translate what they said into her own voice. Moreover, she could remember only her own voice in a conversation: "Sometimes I can extrapolate the other half of the conversation from my remembered reaction. I am immune to what other people say. It's as if their words have lumped and stuck together like porridge while they talk. I just can't get the lumps apart to understand them. Instead I chatter on about goodness knows what, based on my own mistaken assumptions." Sharon reported that other people also found it hard to make sense of her conversation since they often asked for clarification. In retrospect, she could see that she left out facts or else gave too much minute unnecessary detail. Sometimes she realized that she went off on tangents and strayed from the point she was trying to make.

All these difficulties in social discourse had to be kept separate from Sharon's desire for social interaction. She had no wish to be a loner or a recluse. She always craved affection and attention. She was in love with her husband and had a warm relationship with him. She loved her child and enjoyed the company of her few close friends. She had trouble making acquaintances, that was true, but if others were persistent and could see beyond her social gaffes, they were rewarded with her deep and abiding affection. All her life, she had longed for human companionship but had found it only at age fourteen with her first friend, still a friend today, and with people who appreciated her deeper self.

This certainly fit with the kinds of social difficulties I had seen and read about in adults with AS and very high-functioning autism. Eventually such individuals desire social interaction and friendship even though they might act otherwise, particularly as young children. But the desire for attention and affection grows with maturity. I had seen many times the divide that Sharon described between what she desired in terms of relationships and what was observed and experienced by others. It was like a fault line running through the experience of the self.

It was remarkable to me that Sharon was describing exactly the kinds of difficulties in TOM that people with ASD demonstrate. But what was different in her case was that she had such exquisite insight into her own difficulties. People with autism and AS lack a theory of their *own* minds as well as the minds of other people. Sharon was acutely aware of her own lack of understanding, and this was inconsistent with what is usually experienced by people with ASD. Many children and adolescents with ASD are unaware of the way they come across to other children, how and why they are perceived as eccentric by others, and what they do to sometimes irritate their parents and siblings. They also have trouble putting into words how they feel, why they were motivated to do certain things, and why they felt an emotion in a given situation. But perhaps Sharon's acute insight into her emotional life was true only upon reflection. With the aid of logic and with time for reflection, the social world made sense to her, but not in the heat of the moment. Perhaps she was able to compensate for her lack of a TOM with reason and reflection, but she could not do so at an intuitive, preconscious, automatic level. That is the level at which a TOM must operate in the real world. I was beginning to wonder whether Sharon might have a pure and very specific deficit in TOM but was able to maintain her insight and to use her considerable powers of logic to compensate for it to some extent. Perhaps that was the reason for the social rules she had set for herself as an adolescent?

It was also true that Sharon did not appear eccentric to me in the course of the interview. Her conversation was logical, her meaning clear. Yes, she did not always look at me when speaking and did not tend to use gestures to accentuate and emphasize her words, but there was little that was odd or ASD-like in her demeanor. This was perhaps inconsistent with AS in childhood and adolescence. However, in some of the studies our group has conducted, I have seen young adults with AS and even autism (see Chapter 7) whom I had known (or had seen the records of) as children and adolescents and who had shown the same characteristics as Sharon. Observations of the impression she made during the interview were of little help to me in deciding whether or not Sharon might have AS.

It is also true that there are many other reasons that a person might lack a TOM. Sharon clearly was very intelligent—that was readily apparent—and had no difficulty with verbal expression. She did not seem depressed, but a type of anxiety about social interaction was certainly a possibility. The only way to tell was to see if these difficulties in TOM were present at a very early age—or had they perhaps arisen later on in the course of her development? If she had a mild form of ASD, it should be apparent by at least four years of age. If this were a more recent problem, I would have to look for another explanation, like an anxiety disorder. It would also be important to look for evidence of the third part of the autistic triad, the preference for repetitive, stereotyped interests, activities, and behaviors that we saw in Justin and discussed in Chapter 3. If that too were present early on, the evidence for ASD would be strengthened. To obtain this information, it would have been helpful to interview Sharon's parents, but that would not have been appropriate under the circumstances. Sharon felt this would only be distressing to her mother, so we decided to explore her early history from her own perspective. We scheduled a couple of appointments in the next few weeks to go over this information in detail.

*   *   *

Sharon has little memory of the faces of people that were important to her as a child. She is aware of her mother's presence only through the memory of her feet beyond the table on the carpet. She does not remember her grandmother's face, only her hands potting plants in the gardening shed, making a pie crust, sewing, and knitting. She never sees her mother's or grandmother's face, but only their hands and bodies. She remembers their faces only from photographs. In contrast, typical babies will preferentially pay attention to a human face within days of birth. Was Sharon describing the inner experience of lack of eye contact so commonly seen in children with ASD?

She does remember having one or two friends from her neighborhood before kindergarten, but then none until her teenage years. As a young child, Sharon hated physical affection and would struggle to free herself from the hugs of her parents and grandparents. She was lonely, painfully aware of her difference from other children, and confused about why nobody liked her. At one point she realized that she was trying so hard for people to like her that she was making a fool of herself. One time she tried to tell a funny story, but somebody would always interrupt her. She would start again, and again be interrupted. This went on for some time—she might try to tell the story ten or eleven times, not realizing that nobody wanted to hear it. The other girls were just egging her on. But she only realized this as she lay in bed at night going over the day's social fiascoes. Then she would become mortified by the experience. It was hard for her to start a social interaction and even harder to alter her behavior once she got going. She would get stuck in a particular way of responding and could not use the feedback from her peers to be more socially adept. She could not learn the rules of the social game, which were becoming more complex with each passing year.

It was clear to me that these social difficulties were indeed long-standing and were present from an early age. Sharon's problems were clearly of a cognitive nature; they did not fluctuate with her mood. She was not depressed; no mood disorder was clouding her ability to evaluate accurately social interactions. Admittedly, she was anxious in social situations, but the difficulties ran deeper than that. It sounded like a complex cognitive problem, one that was embedded in the spontaneous matrix of peer interactions. If she *thought* about it, she knew what to do. It was at the level of social *intuition*, at a preconscious level, that Sharon was having difficulty with making friends. If it were a simple matter of logic, she would have had no trouble. But her powers of logic were not available to her on the schoolyard. The to and fro of social intercourse was too fast for such leisurely contemplation. She did not feel the complex emotions of guilt, humiliation, and embarrassment in the schoolyard when the event occurred, when she was teased or rejected. It was only in bed at night, under the excruciating microscope of her logic, that she felt these emotions, when she realized with the blinding clarity of reason that she had been made a fool of in front of the very people she wanted to impress most.

There were also other stories from her experiences as a child that were analogous to the experiences of children with ASD and that were consistent with the third element of the autistic triad, the preference for repetitive, stereotyped activities with a high sensory or physical component. Sharon's earliest and most vivid memories are of objects, fascinating in their exquisite visual detail: the patterns in a rug and in her mother's paisley skirt, the sunlight falling on the linoleum floor of her grandmother's house. She has a vivid memory of making candles in the kitchen with her mother but can remember only the different colors of wax dripping down the candle. Sharon always had a penchant for drawing and had an exceptional ability to draw imaginative scenes in perspective at a very early age. She also developed a fascination with several different objects or activities throughout her childhood. The first that she can recollect is a fascination with stones. On her way to school each morning she became intrigued with a patch of gravel. She spent long periods of time staring at the stones, marveling at their brilliance. Sharon might be late for school and knew she would get into trouble, but still the stones held her attention. It was the way they looked, lying there in a dizzying array of patterns. She started to take them home and place them on her shelf, but in that setting they demanded more and more attention. Soon the stones became an irresistible attraction: She felt drawn to them on the way to school, and they appeared to take control of her attention. Eventually she had to take a different route to avoid that patch of gravel altogether.

After the stones, she developed an intense interest in reading novels—or, more precisely, science fiction. These stories held her interest, not the usual stories of romance, action, and adventure that other children might prefer. On the way to school and alone in her room, she dreamt up science fiction plots, endlessly elaborating one or two story lines over and over again, embroidering them but never changing the essential outline. This fantasy soon took over her mind, much like the gravel patch, till she felt a compulsion to fantasize about aliens landing on earth and taking revenge against the children who had been mean to her. She also went through a period of being fascinated with stuffed animals, long after it would have been appropriate. She never played with them; she just placed them on her bed till there was no room left for her. She also experienced compulsive physical urges that were difficult to control. For example, she would rock repetitively, particularly when no one else was there to reprimand her. Even now she feels that she is preoccupied with design—with lines, rectangles, and squares. She cannot avoid thinking about them; such patterns are intrusive and loud, especially when she is trying to talk to someone at the same time. She finds it hard to have a conversation and to see the patterns simultaneously.

These particular experiences of Sharon's cannot be explained by deficits in TOM alone, but they are very reminiscent of the difficulties that children with autism have in executive function and in disengaging attention from the physical world, as described in Chapter 3. These are the types of repetitive stereotyped behaviors and the restricted range of interests that are so characteristic of the disorder and may arise from weak central coherence or difficulties disengaging attention from objects that catch one's interest. Sharon described other types of lapses in attention, but usually in a social context. "I could never maintain a narration or any form of conscious control over my language use while another person was present," she said. She could always be alert and focused in the presence of physical objects, but this sense of awareness would leave her whenever she came in contact with another person. She simply could not focus her attention on people without considerable effort and then only momentarily. She felt like she was in a fog, not part of the real social world. What held her attention were the stones, the stuffed animals, the science fiction fantasies, and, more recently, problems of design. "I made a conscious decision to feel the world in a sensory way, to focus on the now. I craved alertness." I thought her metaphor of being in a social fog was very evocative. Only when the responses of others were very pronounced or exaggerated could she see the outlines of a social interaction looming through the fog. It would lift momentarily, then descend again. At these times she had to use her considerable powers of logic to make sense of other people's minds.

* * *

After three of four sessions, I had a lot of information about Sharon but no definitive conclusions. AS can be difficult to diagnose, especially in adults when there is no corroborating information about early child development. To make a diagnosis, I would have to rely on her developmental history and on her present predicament—the same foundation on which all children with ASD are diagnosed. There is no blood test or brain scan that will tell us who has ASD and who does not. In fact, Sharon's story brought up virtually all of the peculiarities that can make diagnosing ASD challenging.

One difficulty that I had with evaluating Sharon was that most of the adults with autism and AS I had seen were much more impaired than Sharon. They had few if any friends as adults, they had tremendous difficulty in finishing high school or college and even more difficulty finding and keeping a job. In spite of having many symptoms of AS, Sharon showed remarkably little impairment. She had completed high school, gone to college, and graduated with a degree in architecture. She ran a successful business. She was happily married and was raising a perfectly normal and happy boy. She had friends and got along reasonably well with her family (well, at least as well as most people). Sharon had the symptoms but not the impairment. Was it possible to have one without the other? Could one have a pure deficit in TOM without a diagnosis of ASD? She had exquisite insight into her own problems in inferring the mental states of others. Did this insight allow her to develop compensatory mechanisms to overcome her difficulties? And did these compensatory mechanisms leave her with some AS symptoms but not the impairment?

This possibility does raise two important points. The first is that a difference exists between symptoms and impairment. These often go hand in hand, but on occasion there is a marked disjunction between the two. There are some individuals with ASD who are quite impaired but have few symptoms . These individuals may have a later age of on-set and may not have as many repetitive, stereotyped behaviors, because they either are quite developmentally delayed, are very young, or have what some consider true atypical autism. Other individuals with atypical autism tend to be higher functioning, to have some transient language delay but few repetitive, stereotyped behaviors. Because of their language problems, though, they still have a lot of difficulty communicating with others or doing well at school. Alternatively, there are other individuals who have many symptoms but manage quite well in the real world. This latter group tends to keep their eccentric interests to themselves or else share them with friends who have similar interests. These individuals have learned the difference between private and public and keep their eccentricities to themselves. They may go into their room after school and spend hours flicking small plastic tubes, staring at the reflections of a magic lantern on the wall (much like the child narrator, Marcel, in *Remembrance of Things Past*), or echoing conversations heard at school. Like Sharon, they recognize that they are different and take steps to minimize the impact of their symptoms on their functioning in the real world. Perhaps these symptoms are less severe in the sense that the person is able to exert some control over them. Many highly successful adults with autism or ASD are unable to lose their symptoms but are able to function quite well. In fact, I doubt that we can completely eliminate the symptoms of ASD through treatment—the lack of gestures and facial expression, the interests in unusual subjects. But we can help people with ASD improve their social skills, their communication skills, their ability to go to school and hold a job. People with ASD can go a long way in reducing their level of impairment, but they may not be able to entirely lose their symptoms.

The second point is that some of the skills that Sharon used to compensate for her difficulties in TOM could be used by other higher-functioning adolescents and adults with ASD to similar effect. In fact, there is a study showing that children with autism who were specifically taught a TOM were able to improve their ability to correctly assess others' mental states. The skills they were taught were very similar to the compensatory mechanisms that Sharon had come up with on her own. She used her powers of logic and reason to monitor her social behavior and to set up rules for social interaction, to scan what was not appropriate under the circumstances. She used her insight, her memory, her reason, and her ability to think things through to navigate the social world. However, this study also showed that the newly acquired skills did not generalize to everyday encounters. Strategies are needed to take these skills out of the laboratory setting and into the real world. The skills have to be learned over and over again in different situations. Sharon had also developed other compensatory mechanisms that might be helpful in accomplishing this generalization. She used her strengths in visualization to conceptualize her emotions and to organize her day. In a similar fashion, Carol Grey, a teacher who has developed helpful strategies for children with ASDs, has described how social stories delivered in a visual format are a useful way of teaching social skills to young children with autism. Sharon kept to a routine and a structure to maintain order and reduce anxiety. What symptoms she had, she tried to keep private, aware that others would find her interests weird. She repeated others' conversation to herself in order to understand the meaning and context of conversation. In essence, she used her strengths to compensate for her difficulties; she did not practice what she found hard because when she did, it made little difference. Most important, she was motivated to improve her social skills, and this was a key factor in her development. Developing these coping skills takes much effort, and the person with autism or AS must be motivated to learn them. Unfortunately, many people with ASD lack this motivation or find the effort too strenuous. Clinical experience suggests that the timing of the intervention must be absolutely right and works best when individuals are keenly aware of their difficulties and want to narrow the gap between themselves and peers. It also helps to break the social skill down to its component parts and practice each one in turn so that the task does not seem so onerous. Perhaps that is one of the reasons that behaviorally based approaches are so successful; they decompose a complex behavior into smaller and more manageable bits.

*   *   *

These ideas about social interventions apply to high-functioning people with ASD who have some self-awareness and are motivated to improve their social skills. Different techniques are required for younger children who are not as advanced developmentally. Several different programs have been developed that aim to improve social interactions of children with ASD. These differ with respect to their theoretical orientation and the techniques employed to bring those goals to fruition. The interventions can be broadly conceptualized as behaviorally based or developmentally based.

In a behaviorally based approach, an adult systematically teaches simple social skills to a child with autism using trial and error with rewards for successful completion of a skill. These simple skills could include eye contact, orienting to one's name being called, coming to sit near the therapist, learning to take turns, and so on. The idea is that on the basis of these simple skills, more complex social skills can be taught in a similar fashion, though the teaching sessions will eventually have to involve interactions with other adults and typical peers.

The developmental approach starts with a careful assessment of the child's current social skills, places those in a developmental context, and proceeds to set up situations that allow the child to gain skills at the very next level. It is less systematic and more naturalistic in that social interactions are often initiated by the child, with the therapist promoting further development and interaction. Sometimes typical children can be taught to act as therapists to the child with autism and so promote more appropriate social interaction in an inclusive setting. Both these approaches have been found to be successful, though which is most effective is not known because they have never been compared head to head. It is also probably true that characteristics of the child will influence the response to treatment. One can imagine that more developmentally delayed children will respond better initially to the behavioral approach, whereas higher-functioning children can perhaps proceed more directly to the developmental approaches. These can often be implemented in community settings with specialized help. In any case, structure, routine, and appropriate expectations based on the child's current social and communication skills are essential in any treatment approach. To divorce social skills from systematic attempts to improve communication and play skills will reap fewer benefits, and time must be devoted to treating all components of the autism triad.

* * *

In the end, I could not give Sharon a diagnosis of AS. To qualify for that diagnosis there has to be substantial impairment. Sharon's insight into her own predicament was just too good and her accomplishments too impressive. However, there were two other possibilities worth considering. One of the findings of the genetic research in ASD is that some of the relatives of children with autism themselves have ASD-like traits that fall short of a diagnosis. Parents sometimes report that they are, or a more distant relative is, socially awkward, with difficulty initiating and maintaining friendships or being empathic and intimate with others. Some relatives even develop intense interests in esoteric subjects such as astronomy, census data, election results, or computers and math problems, hobbies that occupy them to the exclusion of other family activities. It was conceivable that Sharon had these traits, although there was no family history of autism among her relatives. What she described to me was certainly analogous to the experiences of people with ASD. We know that these traits exist in the general population, perhaps as frequently as five to ten percent. It may be that the genes that give rise to autism are not all that uncommon in the general population. Maybe the symptoms of all the ASDs appear along a continuum and that subclinical cases—those without true impairment in functioning— exist in the general population. Perhaps as these ASD-like traits become more severe, the capacity for insight diminishes as well, until a certain threshold is crossed, or a level of impairment is reached, and a diagnosis of ASD is made.

Another possibility was that Sharon had had AS as a child but had now recovered to such an extent that, even though she might have some symptoms, she did not have any associated impairment. Some people with AS and autism do recover to a remarkable extent (see Chapter 7), though it is, admittedly, uncommon. I have followed some children with AS from early childhood (where it was clear they had an ASD) into adolescence and adulthood. Some of the children with AS (about twenty percent) were functioning in the average range on their social and communication skills, though in private they still might engage in repetitive, stereotyped behavior. Perhaps Sharon was one of these people with AS who was able to "recover" to a remarkable degree?

The existence of ASD-like traits among the general population also gives us an opportunity to realize that maybe ASD is not an all-or-none phenomenon. Perhaps some ASD-like traits are present in all of us, though for a variety of reasons and at different times in our development. It is a humbling thought, but it does encourage us to appreciate the precious opportunity that empathy and having a theory of other people's mind gives us and the obligation it entails. Being socially competent carries a responsibility to do some good in the world. It is not something that is given once and for all but a skill that needs to be affirmed and continuously rehearsed during the traffic of human discourse. From time to time, we all experience the fault line in our natures that separates what we intend to do from what we actually do— what we say in the heat of the moment and what, upon reflection, we wished we had said. But unlike people with ASD, we have a choice, and with that choice comes the responsibility to perform many small acts of kindness.

* * *

I set up a final appointment with Sharon and shared these thoughts with her. In fact, she agreed with these two possible explanations of her difficulties. I believe she was relieved to have a name for her predicament and that whatever possibility was the right one, it did not constitute a "true" disorder (even though she might have had one as a child). Once some complex human problems have a name, the magnitude of the burden diminishes. I had given her a language for her predicament. But she had given me something more important: the language to understand the inner world of people with autism and AS. I do not think it was a fair trade, to be sure. I was in her debt, but I hoped that her initial act of courage in sending that letter had not been in vain. As I said good-bye, my eye happened to catch the lilac tree outside my window. I went out to see if the afternoon mail had arrived, in hopeful anticipation of other gifts that might come my way.

Chapter 6

William
A World without Metaphor

William is very tall and very thin. He wears a blue sweatshirt, blue jeans, and a white turtleneck. The sweatshirt has a logo of a
cartoon character, Sailor Moon, on it. William is fourteen years old and
is visiting me today because his parents are worried he might be depressed. They report that he spends a lot of time in his room, asks the
same set of questions over and over again, and generally appears more
anxious and withdrawn than usual. I notice his long, finely tapered fingers and his clear, almost blue fingernails. He is as delicate as an antique
China vase. William looks down at the carpet, a posture that accentu-
ates his long eyelashes. He rarely looks at me during our conversation.

I try to find out if William is depressed. The difficulty is that he
prefers to talk about other things. "How are you today?" I ask politely.

"I saw the round doors going east at 8:50," he replies.

"I beg your pardon, I missed that," I answer. "The round doors of
what?"

"The subway train," he informs me. Now I understand. William
has always loved the subways. He has memorized the subway map of
Toronto and knows the names of all the stations, what color they are,
and in what direction the trains travel from station to station. Since
there are over fifty stations in the system, that is quite an accomplishment. Every Saturday for years, he and his father traveled the subways
as a treat. William would sit in a seat by the window and look at all the
stations going by, the people coming in and out, noticing the individual

79

decor of each station and each change in direction of the train. He travels the subways by himself now and experiences the same joy and pleasure.

"I remember that you like subways. Can you tell me why?"

"The way they look, the way the doors open and close, the way the trains move. I like the Royal York station because that's where you get a certain kind of door. There is a new subway on the Young–University line." He tells me all this as if I am as interested as he. He begins to talk faster and with much animation as he describes this new line. For the life of me, I can't get him to talk about being depressed. I try a simpler tack and ask him about school: "What did you do at school yesterday?"

"Math."

"What else?" I ask, trying to get him to elaborate.

He pauses briefly, then starts out again: "Last week I took the subway south from Davisville to Bloor. That is what came when I was going to Bloor and Lawrence, at the Royal York to Bloor line in the subway going east. Then we walked to Pamela's place. Then because John was getting T-shirts, I would not leave there until I saw the round doors going west. Because I wanted to catch them when they came east. And I saw one going west at three-thirty-five." The speech comes in waves—slow and strained when talking about his day, fast and animated when talking about the subways. He refers to people I do not know, clauses have ambiguous references, and unexpected words pop up frequently.

William never looks at me to see if I understand. His long, thinly tapered fingers rest easily in his lap as he pretends to roll something. His cheeks are flushed. I tried several times in that interview to steer the conversation back to the issue of depression but without success. It was not that he was avoiding an emotionally laden or uncomfortable topic. I could not even get William to talk about neutral subjects such as the weather or school or sports. The closest I could come to the issue of depression was music. His mother told me that William had developed a fondness for the songs of George Hamilton, especially the ones about heartache and loneliness.

"I understand you like George Hamilton. How come?" I ask, trying not to sound incredulous. William briefly tells me that listening to these songs makes him feel better. But then he quickly returns to the trains at the Royal York Station. For the most part, I have very little idea what William is talking about and I easily become confused between trains going in every direction. The conversation is a vortex of colors, shapes, and times. William cannot help me out. I do not even think he knows I am as confused as I am. In spite of this difficulty in carrying on a conversation, it's remarkable that his grammar and vocabulary are excellent; he uses past tenses appropriately, his sentence construction is perfect—in fact, there is nothing wrong with the more formal aspects of his language. Yet I don't have a clue what he is talking about. There is slippage between the words and the communication. The philosopher Ludwig Wittgenstein wrote that the meaning of language is a function of the "language game" in which it occurs, a function of the context of communication in social discourse. Words have no meaning outside their use. I know we are playing a language game, only the rules are William's own invention and he either won't, or can't, share them with me.

* * *

I first saw William when he was four years old, some ten years ago. His parents asked me to give them a second opinion about his diagnosis. Along with his medical records, they brought in a diary they kept when he was an infant. The delight and joy they experienced as parents fairly jump off the page. Each accomplishment is recorded with pleasure and pride. "William sat up today," "William took his first steps today," "William pulled my hat down over my eyes and laughed." One entry at eighteen months mentions that when the family was traveling in the car, he insisted on going to their usual station to buy gas rather than a new one, even though the new one was much more convenient. Reading the document, I searched for other hints and clues of early signs of ASD but found only the missing bits as potentially ominous. There was no mention of gestures or imitation, pointing or showing things of interest to his parents. No words appeared until eighteen months and no phrases until two years. There was no mention of seeking out other children with whom to play. This inclination to play by himself was brought to the parents' attention by the nursery school staff when William was three years old. They recommended an assessment be completed as soon as possible. The first diagnosis by a pediatrician was autism, but this did not fit with the parents' perception of what a child with autism was like, so they sought a second opinion.

I saw him a little later. At that time, he was able to talk fluently but showed little inclination to do so. He seemed to understand everything his parents said to him, and he would point without any difficulty but still did not use gestures to communicate. There were also some examples of impairments in social reciprocity. He would smile at his parents, was cuddly, would come for comfort when hurt, and was upset when separated from his mother. But with other adults, he would not smile, he avoided their gaze, would look at people from the side, and often hugged other children inappropriately. His social interactions with other children were, in fact, largely limited to playing with his train set and allowing them to sit nearby. It was much more difficult to engage him socially in other play activities.

At age four, there was still no evidence of imaginative play. William was very interested in toy trains and could play with them for hours, but the play consisted largely of repetitive movements of the cars, back and forth, without elaborating a story or making the tiny figurines get on and off the train. He loved to watch the water in the dishwasher, and even as young as age four he loved to travel on the subways, often re-marking on the color of the doors. Later, in elementary school, he be-came intensely interested in elevators and especially the escalators in the subway stations. All the doors in the house had to be open, and he would sometimes walk down the hallways at school backward, presum-ably imitating the sensation of riding in a subway car. Cognitive testing done on a number of occasions consistently demonstrated that he was quite bright, had good nonverbal memory and motor skills, good word recognition and single-word comprehension skills, but more difficulty with complex comprehension of language and problem-solving tasks. If he had to tell a story from a picture or provide a solution to a puzzle, he would not be able to come up with an appropriate answer.

This developmental history is fairly common among children with AS, a type of ASD that differs from autism in a number of ways. Age of onset is often somewhat later, and the social impairments are similar to, but less severe than, those in autism and are usually more apparent in interaction with peers than with parents. Children with AS can speak fluently and usually have age-appropriate grammar and vocabulary, but, much like children with autism who are able to speak, they have signifi-cant difficulties using language socially. Children with autism have sim-ilar problems communicating socially, but they also demonstrate delays in vocabulary and grammar as well. Finally, children with AS have in-tense, often bizarre interests and preoccupations that are somewhat more complex and involved than in autism.

Asperger was a Viennese pediatrician who wrote a paper on "autis-tic psychopathy" in 1944, the year after Leo Kanner's classic paper was published. Both authors borrowed the term "autism" from Eugen

Bleuler, a Swiss psychiatrist who had published a very influential book on schizophrenia some years earlier. Bleuler argued that "autism," defined as a persistent withdrawal from reality, was one of the cardinal symptoms of schizophrenia. Kanner and Asperger believed that the impairments in social interaction seen in the children they were describing were similar to the "autism" seen in schizophrenia. But Asperger used the term "psychopathy" to argue that this was a feature of the child's personality, not an illness like schizophrenia. He did not acknowledge Kanner in his article, suggesting that the two had arrived independently at a similar description. The group identified by Asperger were all verbal, whereas of the eleven children Kanner wrote about, only five were fluent. These fluent children closely resembled the children described in Asperger's paper. This marked the beginning of much overlap and confusion between the terms, a confusion that still exists today.

There has, in fact, been much controversy in academic circles as to whether AS and autism are different disorders. To some extent, this is not a helpful debate. The more important issue is whether it is *useful* to differentiate these two types of ASD. Or should all such children be given the label "high-functioning autism" or "autism spectrum disorder"? Whether or not autism and AS are "really" different requires an understanding of the underlying causes that is well beyond our current knowledge base.

According to DSM-IV, the key differentiating feature between autism and AS is that children with AS "lack clinically significant cognitive and language delays." Children with AS develop speech at roughly the appropriate time; single words are used spontaneously and usefully by around one year, and spontaneous phrase speech with a verb appears by three years of age. The emphasis here is on *spontaneous* and *useful* speech as opposed to *echolalic* speech, which is simple parroting of what another person has said or what the child may have heard on TV. Children with autism may speak early, but the speech is usually echolalic and not spontaneous. One way of thinking about these disorders is to think of autism as AS with an added impairment in language. The differences between autism and AS with respect to their clinical presentation and their outcome perhaps stem from this fundamental difference in language ability. There is also some evidence that children with AS have fewer autistic symptoms and are able to function better in the community than children with autism. However, a subgroup of children with autism can also develop fluent speech, though by definition they do so at a later age than children with AS, between four and six to seven years of age. Once these children develop useful speech they come to resemble more and more the AS children and may eventually catch up to them. On the other hand, both AS and autism appear to arise from a common set of genetic mechanisms. Children with AS can have siblings with autism and children with autism can have siblings (and even parents) with AS. There is also no evidence that treatment needs are any different, though children with autism need speech therapy whereas children with AS are already able to talk. For them, therapy needs to focus on the social use of speech. Therefore, making the distinction between AS and autism may be useful not only in predicting outcome for the child, but also in choosing a focus for treatment.

*   *   *

"And I saw the round doors going east through the windows of the round doors going west. And I saw the round doors going west through the windows of the third coach with gray on the round doors going east. And then I got in the round doors going east."

"Who was with you?"

"Joe and Claire."

"Who are they?" I had heard about Pamela, but not these two.

"My cousin. My three-year-old cousin."

"Who was three years old?" I ask, expecting clarification.

"Then we got downtown at 4:15." I sit back in the conversation, resigned. I must be content to go for a ride, still confused about the meaning of the different shapes and colors. The train is going awfully fast, but I dare not pull the brake handle to slow it down. I have long ago given up asking about depression.

As I listen to William, I realize that I am not part of this conversation. Indeed to even call it a conversation is perhaps inaccurate. I am being talked *at*, not *with*. William and I do not share a common framework, a set of rules, for the creation of shared meaning. As a listener, I experience a profound slippage between what is *said*, which I can perfectly well understand, and what is *meant*, of which I still have no clue. What is *not* being said is as important to the meaning of the conversation as what I hear, but I cannot figure out what that is. I have the sense that there is meaning to this, but it eludes me. I try to project all kinds of meaning onto the torrent of language to imagine what is not said, but none of my conjectures seems to fit. I am, in effect, a passive participant as words are flung at me. I can well imagine how this type of interaction would be very difficult for William's teachers to cope with and how he would be made fun of by his classmates.

William's speech lacks many of the linguistic devices we use to build a conversation. He often will not answer my requests for clarification. He will not repair the conversation when it apparently breaks down. I'm sure he's not even aware that it has broken down. He has little awareness that I need help in following the sense of the conversation. He makes ambiguous references that could refer to several different things or different people but without clarifying the context: What color is he talking about? What shapes? Who was three years old? The topic of the conversation is also not what one might expect. Much of the conversation of typical children involves reference to the social world: Whom did you see yesterday? What was he doing there? In typical conversation, the references are to other people who share the linguistic space of the speaker and the listener. Instead, William refers to the physical world (shapes and colors) with only passing reference to people. He perseverates on trains and returns again and again to the colors, the shapes, and the time of the trains' arrival and their direction, as if I require this information rather than the context of the story. I do not need all these details; I need an overall message.

As it so often does when trying to engage in conversation with a child or an adult with ASD, the sense of it all eludes me. I am immersed in detail, swimming in a whirl of sensations. These familiar words begin to sound strangely unfamiliar. Soon the meaning of individual words starts to slip away. Without an easily identifiable reference, I listen more and more to the sounds and the rhythm of the speech. The constant repetition serves to make the familiar extraordinary.

As I struggle to understand, I can't help wondering if this is the way William feels when listening to other people talk. Does he feel shut out of the conversation, unable to locate meaning in the social use of language? I doubt it, as he shows no distress at my incomprehension and little awareness of my difficulties. No doubt he lacks the insight that Sharon had in her conversations with other people. But William must need to communicate and must enjoy it at some level. Otherwise, why does he tell me all about the subway stations? Most often when children with autism speak it is to ask for something they want, like food, a favorite video, or access to their current interest or preoccupation. Sometimes they will talk about their interests at length, presumably to share that interest with another person. That spark of wanting to share becomes the key to intervention (discussed later in this chapter), but to generalize that beyond the child's interests and preoccupations is very difficult. This situation suggests that some children with ASD want to talk but will not do so in most circumstances (see the story of Gavin in Chapter 1); others cannot talk even with the right motivation and need to rely on augmentative forms of communication such as picture boards and voice boxes.

It also strikes me that William does not use metaphor in his conversation. Things are not *like* something else; they *are* the thing itself. Metaphors are a ubiquitous part of conversation and are an important way of conveying meaning. Many of the concepts and expressions we use have a metaphorical connotation: "Time's a wasting!" "I feel down today." "As I look into the future, I see a bright tomorrow." And so on. The wonder of language is its limitless capacity to convey new meanings. Paradoxically, this is accomplished with a finite number of words and a finite way of combining them using the rules of grammar. To create and understand metaphor is an important linguistic skill that appears to be hard-wired in the brain. Children begin to appreciate metaphors as young as three years of age and can understand the difference between literal and metaphoric meaning as young as five. From an early age, then, metaphors bring coherence to the myriad sensations experienced by us all. It's true that people with autism and AS may use phrases that sound like metaphors. For example, Justin (Chapter 3) would often use clichés, which are really "dead" metaphors: "That sound does not turn my crank anymore," he would say. In this context, he was using "my crank" as a metaphor for a mood state. But it is not a metaphor as I mean it here, because Justin did not come up with it himself to create a new meaning; he only adopted it from common parlance to reiterate an old message. It is no more truly metaphorical than using the literal words to express the same thing. Another type of false metaphor consists of made-up neologisms or words with private and idiosyncratic meanings. These may be interpreted as metaphors by the listener but do not function in this manner for the person with autism or AS. For example, some children with ASD refer to family friends by the cars they drive or by their street address. "Hello, Chevy van," one boy said to a family friend who had just arrived for a visit in his car, a Chevy van. "When is 42 coming for dinner?" another boy with autism asked. In this context, "42" happens to be the street number at which that person lives. In a neologism, some aspect or detail associated with the person becomes that person. The person is effaced by a detail. That detail does not symbolize the person as in a metaphor; it is as if that person *is* the detail. At least that is how it is experienced by the person on the outside of that private meaning.

I remember William once going through a period of calling all men who visited the house "Mr. Pipes." His mother told me that once he saw an anatomical drawing of the inside of a person with the trachea and lungs highlighted. Since seeing that picture he called all men "Mr. Pipes."

"Oh," I said, "it's like they are made of pipes as in the picture."

"No," he said, "they are Mr. Pipes." In other words there was no appreciation that the picture was a metaphor—that people might look like they have pipes inside them but these were drawings used to represent lungs. To William, people had pipes, people *were* pipes, pure and simple.

* * *

Metaphor creates new meaning by allowing us to experience and understand one thing in terms of another. New meaning is conveyed by an unfamiliar combination of familiar words. As a result, metaphors also play a fundamental role in our understanding of the world by structuring language, thought, feelings, and actions and making possible an understanding of complexity, subtlety, and nuance. But children with autism and AS live without metaphors, not only in their language but in their understanding of the world. Living without metaphors is a common theme that runs through many of the cognitive models we've been exploring to explain the symptoms and behaviors of children and adults with ASD—theory of mind, executive function deficits, and weak central coherence (though perhaps not the concept of difficulty in disengaging visual attention). Living without metaphors means there is no distinction between the literal and the figurative; all is literal meaning. Holding two meanings in place at the same time is just not possible. One thing is not understood in terms of another; it is just understood as it is. A facial expression does not imply an emotion, a figure does not imply a ground, a solution that does not work does not imply that one must look for another.

Living without metaphors may be sufficient for many things in life—going to school, turning on the TV, or going shopping—the instrumental demands of daily life. But it is insufficient for the more complex demands of learning, for navigating the ambiguity of social interactions, for self-reflection, and for generating novel ways to solve

problems. Metaphors play a crucial role in each of these important activities. Teachers rely on models all the time to explain things in school;
the solar system is more than a simple mobile strung together with
wires, as one child with autism once explained to me in wonder. We
also think of our social interactions in terms of metaphor. When a
mother said that somebody "got out of the wrong side of bed this morning!" another child with AS asked whether he had hurt himself. We
often use metaphors to creatively solve problems, but a phrase such as
"life by the inch is a cinch, life by the yard is hard" was of no help what-
soever in helping a teenager with AS prepare for tests at school by
studying a little bit each night. Without recourse to these metaphors,
experience cannot by synthesized, integrated, and made meaningful except in the particulars.

To live without metaphor is to live in the particular, without the capacity to generalize experience and to anticipate solutions to new problems, to realize that what is hidden (be it an emotion, a context, or a
general, abstract rule) gives meaning to what is present, makes sense of
the stream of perception. Without the capacity for metaphor in a more
general sense, people with ASD rely on black-and-white rules to govern
behavior, and routine and insistence on sameness to structure their
world. Living in the particular has its own rewards to be sure, but it
does come at a cost.

The poet Wallace Stevens wrote that reality is a cliché from which
we escape by metaphor. Perhaps this is because a metaphor carries a
surplus of meaning—that is, both a literal and a figurative meaning. The
figurative meaning emerges from an implicit understanding of context
by both speaker and listener. Meaning for typical children arises from a
mutual, almost implicit and preconscious understanding of the social
world that encompasses both speaker and listener. What happens in
ASD is that the literal meaning by itself, so often divorced from the context, looks nonsensical to the outsider. To refer to Uncle Bob as "Mr.
Pipes" makes no sense unless the listener can infer a context on *behalf
of* the child. The figurative meaning in this case emerges from the context of the child's interests and his preoccupations (that is, plumbing).
But without knowledge of the special interest, the phrase spoken by the
child with ASD is often meaningless.

The key to helping children with ASD is that as listeners we have to
infer the context: We have to say what is unsaid; we have to supply the
surplus meaning on behalf of the child. We have to drag it out into the
light of day. To accomplish this, we have to put ourselves in the child's

shoes, see the world from his perspective, be aware of the child's interests, concerns, and recent experiences. With this knowledge, an understanding of behavior and communications is much easier. Without it, the potential for misunderstanding grows and can lead to conflict, to challenging behavior, aggression, and "being stuck" in maladaptive and repeated responses.

A simple but common example illustrates this paradigm. A child drags his mother by the hand to the fridge but does not say what he wants or even point to the fridge. If the mother does not infer the child's motivation (that he wants something to eat or drink), the child becomes upset, may start to cry or even hit his mother or himself. Once the mother opens the fridge, having "read" the child's mind, she has to infer again what it is he wants. But it can be only a guess since he cannot, or does not, communicate with her. What are his favorite foods? Has it been a while since he had something to drink? Might he be thirsty instead of hungry? The mother again has to infer a desire on behalf of the child who cannot communicate on his own. If her inferences are wrong, temper tantrums, aggressive behavior, and frustration will follow.

This simple example can be expanded to include a whole range of other situations, at home, at school, or in the community. The most challenging situations are those where the child is quite verbal and, on the surface at least, can communicate quite well. It's easy for parents and others to forget that what is being said is often not what is meant, as in the case of William and the subway cars. I remember one child who, when he got mad, would say the most horrible things to his father, like how he was going to cut him up, disembowel him, and feed him to the birds. Of course the parents were terrified, particularly as he got older and bigger. They were worried that he could become violent and might act on these sentiments. But they needed to realize that he was simply angry and had no more appropriate ways of expressing that frustration. There was no middle ground to his emotion; he either sounded "violent" or was placid; there was no in-between. If they reacted with anger or anxiety, that only made him more frustrated and more violent in his threats. The key was to recognize that he did not mean what he said, react calmly, respond to the real message that lay behind the threats, and try to teach him more appropriate ways of expressing his frustration. Once they started calmly ignoring the threats and saying things like "You must be upset. Are you upset? Tell me that you are upset. Now tell my why," the threats diminished over time. They realized that their anxiety only increased their son's frustration, which made matters that much worse.

The same thing can happen in school with teachers who don't know the child as well as the parents. Too often teachers react to the overt behavior or communication of the child and don't look behind to the context, the recent history, to understand the child. The most effective form of behavior management in schools is to actively "read the mind" of the child with ASD and not assume that what is said or expressed is what is meant. Before the teacher tries to "manage" the behavior, it's imperative to understand what it means. If the teacher does not know the child well enough, parents can often provide that information quickly and efficiently. That's why it is so important that parents and teachers work together as a team. Too often, teachers and parents eye each other suspiciously across the table and cannot form a partnership to provide that context for the child's communications. The parents have to teach the teacher how to read their child's mind. In that way, understanding becomes possible and the transition to school that much easier.

*   *   *

Finding the right context that day with William was a matter of trial and error. I tried out various contexts to understand his kaleidoscope of color and shape but came up empty. On other occasions it was easier, because once William was aware I was having a hard time, he could help me repair the conversation by supplying answers to my questions. With William, once the background was explicitly clarified between us, dissonance could be reduced, and meaningful contradictions might emerge. Then Mr. Pipes seemed quite appropriate as a description of Uncle Bob, the "weekend handyman." One reason I was having particular trouble that day understanding William was that the references to a shared context were cut and meaning flew where it might, determined only by his interests, independent of the context or the needs of the listener. Even though I had a good appreciation for his interests, his worries, and his recent life experiences that might constitute a context, I suspect his mood was getting in the way of his ability to help me understand the particular context operating in the background of our conversation.

*   *   *

"And then the brownish going north went into Bloor and then the yellowish going south came into Bloor. And I saw the brownish go north through the windows of the yellowish going south. And I let the yellowish going south go by."

"You let another one go by?"

"And then it went into a tunnel. And then you know what happened?"

"No."

"The yellowish going south came in all over again!"

"I imagine you were quite late getting home."

"And then the brownish going north came in again. And I saw the brownish going north through the windows of the yellowish going south. The yellowish going south on that side and the brownish going north went outside. And then the new subway going south came into Davisville. And it had a trip arm sticking out of the front. And the doors are a lot bigger in it."

"Is that good?"

"And there's windows and there is a wheelchair sign on it. That's why the doors are bigger."

"To allow the wheelchairs to go in?"

"No. And then you know what happened?"

"No."

"It stopped, and I let it go by because I wanted brownish. And it left. The new subway going south left Davisville. And the new subway going south went outside. Then the other subway with yellowish going south came into Davisville again."

And then I see! I can finally picture in my mind what is going on. Imagine William's perspective as he stands on the subway platform. He is waiting for a particular train to come in, and he lets other trains go by as he waits for the right one. The "right" train is a particular combination of direction, shape of window, and color of upholstery. He sees various trains come into the station, some with square windows, some with round windows. Some trains have yellow upholstery, some have brown. He watches as the trains move past each other, one going north, one going south. Through the square windows of one train going north he sees the round windows of the other train going south. It is a kaleidoscope of shapes and colors going in both directions. From William's perspective the entire conversation makes sense. It is no use forcing my perspective onto his conversation. I have to see things just as he does, then I can have a conversation with him. But without that imaginative leap on my part, I understand nothing. I have to see the world as William does. He cannot make that imaginative leap to me; I have to construct a metaphor of his world in my mind and then interpret what he says. Only in this way can we play the same language game. I must have a hypertrophied theory of mind to bridge the gap that separates us. To appreciate the context, I have to see and imagine the world as experienced by William, standing on the platform, waiting for the subway to arrive.

*   *   *

William's parents have asked me on several occasions whether these difficulties in initiating and sustaining a conversation can be improved. I rather reluctantly tell them that very little research has been done on this topic. Speech therapy is certainly an effective form of treatment for very young children with ASD and, in particular, those who are nonverbal and are just beginning to speak and to communicate their needs and wants. But once speech develops, there are no standard interventions that can improve the social use of language in conversation. But having a conversation with William does suggest certain strategies that might be helpful. These are based on the notion that the conversational difficulties of people with ASD are caused by the difficulties in theory of mind, the inability to use certain linguistic devices that are typically used to initiate and sustain a conversation, and by the deficits in executive function and weak central coherence that are so characteristic of children with ASD (see Chapters 4 and 5). It is of no use to try to teach children with ASD the use of metaphor or to have them practice what they can't do. Instead, we can teach them the specific rules they need to get by in conversation with others. Slowly over time, the capacity to hold a coherent conversation with another person improves as the child's social skills improve as well. This usually happens during the teenage years, and it may be worthwhile to hold off implementing some of these strategies until that time.

The intervention consists largely of having a conversation with the adolescent, making sure that a shared context is explicitly present for the conversation and practicing the rules that govern social intercourse. This involves encouraging the child to use certain simple linguistic devices that make conversation coherent. The focus is not on the use of grammar or vocabulary or the meaning of individual words but on the initiation and sustaining of a conversation. The objectives are to help children become consciously aware of the listener's needs in the conversation and to teach them linguistic devices to keep the conversation going.

It's important to first set the parameters of the conversation. Practicing has to be a natural part of everyday life, not seen as a time for "therapy." The conversation must be fun so the child sees the value of engaging in social interchange through conversation, and it should not be coercive but part of the natural flow of the day's routine. The conversation is best carried out by parents, teachers, or older siblings who can understand the new rules of the game or that the language game will have to be played at first by somebody else's rules. It is essential, as my conversation with William demonstrates, that the context be front and center in any conversation with a child with ASD. Techniques to set the conversational context can be established by asking about common events, practicing conversations that might occur on a routine basis with typical children, and talking about a child's special interests. This ensures that a common context is established that allows the speaker and listener to build shared meaning. Discussing common events like finding out what happened at school, how people were feeling, what somebody's behavior was like are especially helpful. It's also useful to make the conversations functional. What conversational abilities does one need to survive in the world, to use change to buy things at the store, to ask for directions, and so on? Practicing going to the store or using the bus can be excellent opportunities to teach these skills and to learn certain routines. Using visual aids can also be helpful—books, pictures, or the TV can be a useful way of facilitating communication and of initiating a conversation.

It is also very effective to initiate a conversation on the child's favorite topic. This will make the context abundantly clear and tends to elicit the most speech and the most appropriate social skills. I try to engage in the conversation on the child's terms for a while but then steer it toward other, more appropriate topics like what happened at school, what it is about a sibling that bugs him the most, and so on. This redirection can be difficult, and it sometimes feels like setting up signposts that are ignored consistently. But persistence eventually pays off.

The key to creating a common context is to realize that sometimes what's being said by the child with ASD is not always what is meant. It's that imaginative leap to the context that the child with ASD is operating from that is often required to make sure the conversation makes sense. I always try to clarify with the child an ambiguous context to make sure we're speaking with a common frame of reference: "Are we talking

about subways here or what Pamela and John saw?" Repetitive questioning is a common problem in conversation and is a good example of
the difficulty in inferring the context from which a child speaks. A child
with autism or AS will often ask the same question over and over again,
even after the appropriate answer is given. Usually there is *another*
question that the child wants an answer to, but he or she cannot disengage from the first topic. The child asks a question arising from a context that's hidden, but parents and teachers often answer from the context that's visible.

I remember one boy who repetitively asked what would happen if
he got in trouble at school. Each time his parents tried to reassure him
that he rarely gets in trouble anyway, he asked the same question right
away. That led to all kinds of problems, sometimes even aggression and
a sense of frustration on the part of both the child and his parents. But
since that wasn't really the child's question, he had to ask it again and
again, in the same way as before. I spent a lot of time trying to figure out
what question he was really asking It turned out he was very concerned
about other children teasing him at school and why *they* didn't get in
trouble for *that* behavior. Once we talked about that issue, the repetitive
questions subsided.

Another example is the little boy who over and over again asked
whether it was time to bring out the Christmas tree, even though it was
the middle of July. His parents would answer that it was much too early.
In fact the little boy was not asking a question, but making a request to
bring out the tree now, whatever the time of year. Once we realized this,
he was taught to make the direct request instead, and as a reward the
parents brought out the tree on the twenty-fifth of each month for a little party. It was a little extra work but paid off in other ways as he
started to ask fewer repetitive questions in general.

Teaching social skills also has a direct impact on conversational
abilities. It may be useful, for example, to try to teach children with autism and AS a theory of mind, to expand their horizon of interests, to
help them not get stuck in the details of a situation. Since those with autism are not intuitively aware that their behavior might have a negative
impact on others, active feedback is required for them to understand
that. I will tell them I have trouble following the train of the conversation or I'm a bit bored and we should talk about something else. I sometimes give the child a visual or verbal prompt to help him generate a
novel response in the conversation or to help him switch topics. This
helps get him "unstuck" and can break the chain of perseveration.

It is also essential to have a good idea of the linguistic tools the child uses, or does not have access to, when engaging in a conversation. What conversational devices does the child employ that are troublesome for other people to tolerate and that need to be limited? What linguistic tools are missing and need to be applied by asking for feedback and clarification? I ask a lot of questions to get around ambiguous references. I try to slow the speech down if it is too fast or speed it up if it's terse and there are long pauses. I frequently interrupt to encourage the child to get to the point and not spend so much time on the details. I will take the physical context that the child refers to and ask about people in that context. This constant feedback teaches adolescents to be more aware of the skills and linguistic devices needed to have a coherent conversation, so they can keep those rules in their head and use them on their own.

*   *   *

Treating the pragmatics of conversation is a matter of gentle persuasion, of challenging the conversation but at the same time being respectful of the child's level of development. It's a process of not asking too much but not being afraid to challenge and expect more than what is usually given, of seeing the world through the child's eyes by taking that imaginative leap but also holding our own world in mind as we gently encourage the child to move from one to the other. If the language game can become more public and less private, more open to a shared context, then the capacity for relationships improves. It is a matter of enticing children with autism and AS to enter our world and show them how much fun it is and then gently closing the door behind them so they don't have to go back into the world of subways going every which way. This type of gentle challenge may give them a choice between the sense of the word and the presence of the world and allow them to go back and forth at will. To live without metaphors is to live among the particulars, to inhabit a tapestry of details, intricate and fascinating in their design. But it is limiting in that the experience cannot be generalized and categorized. Some things are best left uncategorized to be sure. To have the choice to see the myriad detail here, and then to categorize there, must surely be a privileged place from which to experience the world. Would that we all had that talent.

Chapter 7

Teddy
Incongruous Time,
Incongruous Development

*T*he office was more of a mess than usual after the last appointment of the day. I looked around at the scene—my papers were on the floor, books had been pulled from the shelves, crayons had been broken, a new toy truck thrown against the wall, and my coffee cup smashed. All in a day's work, I thought, but this was a bit much. I felt sorry for the parents who had just left and who must have been mortified that four-year-old Teddy had caused such havoc over the last hour or so.

Teddy was very hyperactive and difficult to control since his understanding of language, and of the word *"no"* in particular, was so limited. It had been obvious that he was not behaving this way to get attention or because he was mad. But since he had not yet developed any play skills, he could only amuse himself by watching things move through the air and make a sound as they hit the floor or the wall. He was quite impulsive; a thought came into his mind and he acted on it, regardless of the consequences. I was told that at home he was much the same— jumping on the couch, climbing on tables and shelves, pulling out the pots and pans from the kitchen cupboards. Each night between 4:00 and 6:00 P.M. he would run between the kitchen, the living room, and the dining room nonstop till his ears were red and he was out of breath. His parents, Sean and Melody, had a younger daughter and an older son at home as well. Sean was a salesman who traveled a great deal. Melody did not have family in the area, having moved here from England, and so she had little support to cope with the chaos that sometimes accompanies a child who has both autism and hyperactivity.

Our appointment that day was intended to be a feedback session, where parents ask questions about autism and what it means for the future. The same three questions come up time and again during these sessions: What caused the disorder, what can we expect for the future, and what can we do to help? We had little opportunity to talk seriously that day while Teddy was running around, so I suggested that we meet again without any of the children and talk about what was uppermost in their minds.

When they returned a few weeks later, my heart went out to them. As they came into the office I could see that they were very anxious. I knew that during college Melody had taken a course in psychology and had learned about autism from textbooks that were now out of date. Sean had first heard about autism from movies he had seen on TV. What they knew about the disorder was pretty discouraging.

"In college, I read that institutionalization was common, that children with autism grow up to be loners, they can't live without their parents, they require constant supervision and are never normal," Melody said tearfully, shaking as she presented me with the information that had frightened them both so deeply. While his wife spoke, Sean stoically looked out the window, grim faced. Then he turned to me and said, "All I know is what I've seen on TV: autistic adults sit in a corner all day and rock back and forth, they don't talk to anyone, and they injure themselves when they get mad. Like Rain Man. Is that true? Is that what we have to look forward to?"

As if the floodgates had opened, questions poured forth one after the other as Sean reached over and held his wife's hand tenderly: "Is there any chance he will be normal?" "Do you know of any adults with autism?" "How have they turned out?" I could just imagine them in the kitchen, talking quietly after all the children had been put to bed, eager to comfort each other but finding it difficult to do so, wondering about the darkness that threatened to envelop them in the future.

I did indeed know some adults with autism and proceeded to tell them about Woodview Manor, a supported independent living program for young high-functioning adults with autism and AS.

* * *

Woodview Manor is meant to provide its residents with the skills needed for independent living in the community. It is run by Rick Ludkin, a child care worker who used to work with adolescents who had trouble with the law. He became interested in autism when one adult with ASD that he was helping was inappropriately charged with an offense. That adult turned out to be very rewarding to work with, and Rick developed an entire program to help adults with ASD as a result. Woodview is home to about ten adults with ASD, all of whom are high functioning. They learn to cook for themselves, to budget, to buy food, to do laundry, and generally look after themselves. They also receive some vocational training, and the staff tries to help the residents find jobs. The annual Christmas party at Woodview happens to be my favorite seasonal event. Each year the house is festooned with the usual Christmas decorations, and everybody brings their favorite potluck dish for the buffet meal. I usually bring a curry, which people find slightly exotic but rarely eat. The residents are nicely dressed, in jacket and tie with perfectly pressed pants. They are certainly better dressed than I, and better than many of the staff as well, who are not much older than the residents themselves. I like to bring my wife and children so they can meet the people with whom I work.

I've known a few of the residents for a long time, some as long as fifteen years. I've watched them grow and mature into young adults. The change is quite astonishing, but none of the residents could be considered socially skilled or even normal by the usual standards. They greet me politely, ask my family a standard set of questions, and then leave it to me to continue the conversation. They are somewhat stiff and formal, but I know it takes enormous determination and strength of character to do this much. The residents have been told countless times that they must greet people, that it's the "proper" thing to do. They have a natural inclination to retire, to back away from saying hello. They contend with a type of social inertia that is so heavy it must weigh down on them. To initiate social interaction, to participate in a social ritual is not easy for them, and I can tell they are quite uncomfortable. Nevertheless I'm grateful that they make the effort and see me as a continuing part of their lives, even though I may not be their physician anymore.

I meet their mothers and fathers again each year. We say hello, and I politely inquire how things are this Christmas compared to last. Over time I feel less like a doctor but not quite like a friend of the family. In many cases, I've been present at times of crisis, when one client was suspended from school or another made a suicidal gesture. But I have also witnessed personal triumphs, like graduating from high school and going out on a first date. I walk a difficult line between knowing too much and too little because my clinical perspective on their family life is so limited. Typical teenagers have coaches, teachers, or Scout masters who know them well and who can talk to parents with easy knowledge of their child's personality and temperament. It is perhaps a sad comment that so few high school teachers take an interest in adolescents with ASD that the residents at Woodview Manor have to make do with me.

Of course, as at many Christmas parties, Santa Claus makes an appearance and distributes presents. The residents become incredibly excited. Many shout with glee, some jump up and down and rock back and forth. All of a sudden these formally attired young men and women act like young children. They let down their guard, their carefully constructed social armor recedes, and, for some, the autistic mannerisms, long held in private check, return. One twenty-four-year-old young man starts to repeat "It's Santa Claus. It's Santa Claus" over and over again while rocking back and forth in front of the mirror. You would never catch him doing that under usual circumstances. The effort required to look "normal" is swept away by the excitement of a present from Santa Claus himself. Do they know that Santa is actually Garry Stuart, the executive director of Woodview, and that he does this every year? If they do, this knowledge does not diminish their enthusiasm one bit.

My children are also excited, not only because they too get presents from Santa but also because they can pretend to be his helpers. They put on their elves' caps and assist Santa as he reaches into his bag and pulls out the presents. As each person's name is called out, he or she sits on Santa's knee and answers some inane question before he gives that person a present. Eventually I get called up, to the accompaniment of much hooting and hollering.

"Have you been a good boy this year?" Santa asks me.

I blush and stammer out an equally inane answer. Everybody laughs at the same jokes told year after year as we all participate knowingly in this ritual of gift giving. It is the familiarity that is comforting. Among the residents, though, the sense that this is a game seems to be absent. They are genuinely thrilled to be sitting on Santa's knee and receiving a present from him. At some level, I'm sure, they know that this Santa is not real, that he's an excuse for a party. But their actions tell more about their beliefs; they experience real enthusiasm and joy each Christmas. No jaded comments from them on the commercialization of Christmas. We, on the other hand, are self-conscious when we sit on

Santa's knee. We're aware of the difference between the fantasy and the reality; we know we are playing a game, can be uncomfortable with it, but go along all the same. The residents too know this is a game but are happy and thrilled just the same. Their social naiveté saves them from the cynicism that we so often feel.

What is most astonishing about the whole experience is the opportunity to watch the residents exchange gifts among themselves. This usually occurs during the quiet moments after Santa has finished handing out his presents. There is genuine pleasure in this simple act of exchange. One resident gives another a set of Laurel and Hardy tapes because the recipient so loves these comedians and often replays entire episodes of the films in his mind, scene for scene. Another gives his friend a special edition of *LIFE* magazine filled with photographs from the last decade. The gift is inexpensive, but since the recipient loves magazines and old photos, the present could not be more appropriate. What is astonishing is the thought that goes into the choosing of such gifts. There is no sense of embarrassment that these gifts might be considered eccentric by others or might reflect peculiar tastes. The choice of gift shows a real awareness of the other's interests. Often when I buy a gift I have to be careful not to buy something that I covet for myself. Buying a present for another can be a vicarious way of buying for oneself. For people without a fully developed theory of mind (see Chapter 5), the residents' ability to buy presents that another person will truly appreciate and enjoy is impressive. Given the difficulties in empathy that people with ASD experience, the giving of gifts is a major accomplishment for these residents. These are enormous gains if seen from the perspective of the disorder, but perhaps tiny and insignificant if seen from the view of the uncomprehending public. Is it the same kind of empathy that we feel when we try to think of a present for another person, a loved one? Surely the test of that is the appropriateness of the gift, its success in making the receiver grateful and happy, and in making sure the gift has no hidden strings or is not intended to convey a hidden message. A gift from a person with ASD is simply a gift, nothing more, nothing less. And the simple giving of gifts is surely one of the hallmarks of being truly human.

The contrast between their childlike behavior sitting on Santa's knee and the maturity of adult friends exchanging presents in an atmosphere of genuine intimacy is remarkable. Questions like those raised by Sean and Melody bring up others, of course, about the nature of this seemingly adult behavior. Is this real and genuine intimacy? I decide there's no use asking myself that question. Is it any less real or genuine than the intimacy I feel with my wife and children? How could I ever compare experiences of intimacy, quantitatively or qualitatively? I can only conclude that the intimacy and thoughtfulness that go into the selection and giving of these presents is as deep and as meaningful as it is for typical people, perhaps even more so since there are no hidden messages in these gifts, as there so often are in typical families and relationships. These are true gifts with no strings attached, since to a large extent the capacity to attach strings to gifts is lacking.

I know three of the residents better than the others: Justin (from Chapter 3), Jeremy, and Tom. All three are in their late twenties, early thirties. Jeremy and Tom have AS, and Justin has autism. All three experienced considerable hardship growing up, coping with the academic expectations of teachers and the taunts of other children. Nevertheless, they are all proud of their recent achievements and of living away from home.

Justin loves to listen to music, Tom is an avid reader, and Jeremy likes to walk all over town. They are good friends; they like to spend time together, to talk about their mutual interests, to share experiences just like everybody else. However, being with others is not the only thing in their life; they also like to be alone to pursue their own interests. Tom does not take it wrong if Jeremy does not call him every Friday night to go out on the town.

With each other, they are without guile, incapable of telling a lie or being deceitful, and they are never violent. Neither are they cruel to each other or in the habit of making fun of each other's eccentricities and foibles. These acts, typically seen in normal people, require a sophisticated theory of mind and excellent executive function skills, which are deficient in people with ASDs, as seen in earlier chapters. One has to know what the other person will believe to be able to lie to him successfully. One has to carefully plan a certain course of action and anticipate the reaction of others to be deceitful. Justin, Tom, and Jeremy are innocent of many sins except perhaps sloth; no doubt they would prefer to indulge themselves rather than do work or chores around the house. It is true they are not "normal," if being normal includes the capacity to lie, to deceive, to be cruel to each other, and to humiliate their fellow human beings. Their parents and the staff know that to put them out into the world in an unprotected environment would be like the slaughter of the innocents. Yet they are adults and are definitely part of the community, even though they live on the margins of human relationships and are, by most standards, "antisocial." "What exactly do 'normal' and 'antisocial' mean in this context?" I ask myself each Christmas.

This disparity of abilities, appearance, and human characteristics presents an incongruous picture. In these adult bodies are hidden child-like qualities, yet it's not enough to say their development is arrested. Even young children lie and are cruel to each other, and an adult with autism is not like some modern-day Peter Pan who refuses to grow up and who loves to play children's games instead. It is the incongruity of development that is so very striking.

In some ways, the residents of Woodview are typically adult, in others so innocent and child-like, in yet other ways, quite unique and remarkable. To see them is to be aware of the fracture of time, how we are all made of different lines of development that proceed at their own pace, according to their own timetable. For most of us, the disparate parts of ourselves develop synchronously, like a harmonious piece of music. Our abilities keep pace with our interests, our intellect with our appearance. For people with ASD, each developmental line more or less keeps its own company and the disparate parts develop relatively inde-pendently. More than that, different people with ASD develop in differ-ent ways; there are many developmental trajectories or pathways that ASD children follow as they mature and change over time. Sometimes the music is harmonious, like Brahms, sometimes it is like modern atonal music, all discord and harsh notes, often it is repetitive like Philip Glass, but it is never the silence of John Cage. And each person is his own composition, with his own rhythm and pace, volume and pitch.

I remember experiencing this incongruity or asynchrony most viv-idly when I went to a re-release of *Star Wars* with my children. In the row behind us, a group of distinguished-looking gentlemen sat, well dressed and composed. Most had silver hair or were balding and were attired casually in golf shirts and well-pressed pants. They were not eat-ing popcorn like the rest of us but were quietly talking to each other. For all the world they looked like a group of men in their fifties and six-ties, out to enjoy a kids' movie. Perhaps they were like Trekkies, adults who had made *Star Wars* the center of an interest group. Perhaps they were amateur film critics who like to go to the movies, and afterward, over a cappuccino or two, discuss the cultural implications of *Star Wars* and its derivation from Western civilization's archetypal myths.

Then the movie started. They began whooping and hollering like the rest of us. All of a sudden I realized they were probably residents of a group home for developmentally disabled adults. They were out on the town watching their favorite movie and could hardly contain their glee at all the familiar characters. They laughed at the outlandish space aliens, they hissed at Darth Vader, they were tense when Luke Sky-walker was about to launch his devastating missile. At the end of the show a young woman led the elderly gentlemen out of the theater like obedient children. Here again was time's fracture, its veering off in separate directions. This potential incongruity in our lives is made apparent by the striking contrast of outward appearance and inner life. There is chronological time measured by clocks, and there is personal or lived time, measured by subjective experience. But there is also developmental time, which one becomes aware of only upon seeing its asynchrony in certain biologically vulnerable individuals. It is the incongruity of developmental lines that is so remarkable among adults with autism and AS. We are not made aware of this crack in the surface of time unless there is a fault in nature. Time is always at the heart of the matter.

* * *

"What will happen to Teddy when he grows up?" Melody and Sean look at me expectantly. What can I possibly say to them about the incongruity of time—about the individual tragedies and triumphs of development? I cannot lie to them, but neither can I leave them without hope. The truth lies somewhere between the awful stories Melody read about in college and the overly optimistic pronouncements of definite cures that one reads about on the Internet or in the newspaper. Some children do remarkably well—that is true—better than anyone could have anticipated years ago. But normal? There is no evidence to support that view. How could one ever decide that anyway? And besides, normal is not all it's cracked up to be. Justin, Jeremy, and Tom have some attributes that normal adults don't have. They are gentle, kind, sometimes naive and innocent, and enjoy many simple, but exquisite, experiences in life. I hope my children will grow up with some of these attributes as well. I hope they too can sometimes see without metaphors, can see the patterns and structure of nature, the continuity of lines, whether composed of ants on the sidewalk or vines hanging from a tree or beads suspended from a ceiling. I hope they too can see the infinite variety of white paint in Robert Ryman's works and the infinite variety of thunderstorms that Justin perceives (see Chapter 3). Wisdom is sometimes the capacity to act innocently, and courage is the capacity to act innocently in the face of overwhelming circumstances to the contrary. It takes a perceptive observer to see the wisdom and courage in children and adults who struggle to make sense of the actions and motivations of other people. In a world buzzing with social exchange that takes place at the speed of light, one can only marvel at the adaptations that people with ASD make to survive.

*   *   *

Sean and Melody were well aware that the scientific literature (especially the older literature) on the outcome of children with autism makes for abysmally depressing reading. In the past parents were very likely to hear these prognoses, and unfortunately, this may still happen today. For example, a study published in the 1970s reported that seventy percent of adults with autism were institutionalized during the fifties and even up to the late sixties. Thankfully, this has changed, and most adults with autism live at home or in some kind of supervised setting. Those who are higher functioning can even live alone and look after themselves in some circumstances. In fact, the current literature on the outcome of autism is much more optimistic today given the availability of early intervention and the number of children with milder forms of the disorder who do not have as bad an outcome as the more severely impaired.

Unfortunately, many professionals are still not aware of this new information and have continued to rely on the older, more discouraging, information. This has led to two common scenarios. The psychiatrist that Justin's parents took him to as a child said, "He has autism, and you should make arrangements to have him institutionalized when he grows up." Parents who have heard this kind of pronouncement know how indescribably devastating it can be. Clinicians often justify these comments by saying it's better to make parents face reality than to allow them to hide behind denial. What they are forgetting, however, is that denial is what makes hope possible To deny the future, to choose *not* to see it for now is essential to the process of healing, the mourning involved in coming to terms with the fact that the child you had hoped for, dreamed about, and waited patiently for, is not the one you were given. With the new data on the effectiveness of interventions (both early and during childhood), there is no justification for being so discouraging about the future, especially among the higher-functioning group like those with AS. The psychiatrist that Tom's parents consulted took the second, and currently more common, approach: He delayed giving the diagnosis as long as he could since the clinical presentation was not "classic." He did not know there is no such thing as "classic" autism anymore. The enormous variation in clinical presentation in autism, the fact that the clinical picture changes over time, and the realization that there are other forms of ASD that share some features with autism but may look different is perhaps the most important advance in the science of ASD over the last two decades.

Most parents notice something not quite right with their child's development within the first two years of life. Often, however, they do not receive a diagnosis until five or six years of age. Making a diagnosis earlier is difficult, but we are learning more and more about the very early signs of the disorder. As this new information percolates down from the researchers to front-line clinicians, one can only hope that these delays in receiving a diagnosis can be eliminated. Perhaps the most important finding is that the early diagnosis relies heavily on an assessment of social–communication skills in young children. Toddlers with ASD infrequently show the range of repetitive stereotyped behaviors (rocking, rituals, resistance to change, spinning wheels, etc.) more commonly seen in older children. Too often, the diagnosis of AS does not come until even later, at eight or nine years of age. Family doctors, not yet aware of this new information, try to reassure parents that their initial concerns about social and communication skills in infancy and toddlerhood are the results of too much worrying, of having a first child, or of sheer lack of knowledge about child development. This reluctance to give a diagnosis early on leads to significant delays in getting children into early intervention programs. Some children who start these programs at five or six years of age have less prospect of improvement than if they could start receiving therapy much earlier. There are few more frustrating experiences for parents than to be told first they are too worried about their child's lack of speech and then, two years later, that he has autism but now the waiting lists are too long to receive timely interventions.

Clinicians have tended to overlook the fact that we've had reports of good outcome among some children with autism for decades. Kanner titled one of his last papers "How Far Can Autistic Children Go in Social Adaptation?" In this 1972 paper, he reported on the "best outcomes" among the first ninety-six children with autism seen at his clinic. He identified eleven (out of ninety-six) who he felt " functioned gainfully in society." Indeed, the case studies show remarkable improvement but still demonstrate difficulties in intimate adult relationships. The enormous variation in outcome is perhaps the most striking thing about the adult development of individuals with ASDs. Some (our data would suggest that roughly twenty percent of those with AS and ten percent of those with autism) do very well and score in the "average" range on assessments of social and communication skills and have few, if any, autistic symptoms. Perhaps another fifteen to twenty percent do well enough to live on their own with some support. However, the new generation of children who received early intervention has not yet reached adulthood, so even these estimates may need to be revised upward.

The fact is the majority of children with autism and AS will get better. Each year tends to be better, and less stressful, than the last. The most difficult years are the early ones, when the diagnosis is first given and when all that effort must go into early intervention. But after a while, things settle down and the children follow their own developmental timetable. Different skills will develop at their own rate; sometimes a step backward will be taken, sometimes two steps forward will bring about immense relief. Sometimes, what looks like regression is, in fact, the response to a new challenge that the child is not quite ready to meet but with a little support will be able to accomplish in time.

Where any individual child will end up on the developmental pathway is unknown; no one can predict the final outcome. The accomplishments of a child with ASD will look disappointing only when viewed from the outside, when compared to everybody else's yardstick. "He is not meeting our expectations, I am afraid," Justin's teacher once told his parents, who immediately became extremely discouraged with his progress. But it's much better to look at outcome from the perspective of the child's world. What obstacles did he have to overcome to get this far? What challenges did he meet that we can only imagine? The triumphs of a child with ASD are often private, like persisting in going to school in spite of the constant teasing and bullying, like trying to strike up a conversation in the lunch room with another child, like sharing time on the computer with a brother for the first time. Many of these triumphs are known only to parents, but they are no less real for all that. In typical children's families, these accomplishments are often taken for granted. Parents of children with ASD can take nothing for granted; each step toward "typical development" is a victory and sticks out from the daily flow of life's events like a beacon of shining light. The yardstick to measure success should not be the successes of other children but the child himself, last year or the year before.

One of the things that struck me forcibly when I started working in this field a couple of decades ago was that the outcome literature on autism did not seem to apply to higher-functioning individuals. The published studies were quite old, conducted in the days when autism was felt to be caused by poor parenting. At that time, parents were often enrolled in long-term psychotherapy with a social worker and the child was given years of play therapy. That literature was no longer relevant since it was conducted before the emergence of more effective forms of early intervention based on behavioral principles. However, the newer data on outcome had not trickled down to the general public. Moreover, there were no data on the outcome of the other forms of ASD, like AS. Since many more children were getting this diagnosis, there was a significant gap in the evidence. Could I help fill it?

My first experience with research was a follow-up study I conducted in 1987 in collaboration with the West End Crèche in Toronto. At that time, the Crèche was known as the center where autistic children were treated. The physician in charge was Dr. Milada Havelkova, a Czech anesthetist who had immigrated to Canada after the war. The only job she could get was in child psychiatry, and she was given the Crèche as a clinical base. There she became very interested in autism, and starting in the early fifties, the Crèche became the therapeutic center for these children in Toronto.

I wanted to contact the adults who had been given a diagnosis of high-functioning autism by Dr. Havelkova as children. She was very gracious and enthusiastic about the possibility that her work might be continued. I remember spending one very snowy Christmas Eve day in the basement of the Crèche, going over all the old client files from the early days. I sat in the basement of the old building in what used to be the laundry room. The ancient wringer washer was still there, and there were old files in boxes and cabinets everywhere. It was dusty, damp, and cold. There must have been at least five hundred files that had to be pored over. It was quite revealing to read those old charts, with their antiquated terms (childhood psychosis, brain-damage, symbiotic psychosis), to get a glimpse of Toronto and how special needs children were treated at that time. It was disconcerting to think that while I was growing up in this very city, there were other families living such dramatic and often hopeless tragedies within miles of my house.

I managed to contact twenty adults with autism treated at the Crèche in the '50s who were said to be higher functioning as children and still lived in the city. I traveled to their homes and interviewed them and their parents. What surprised me was how well a small subset of children had done. Of the twenty, four had done remarkably well; they were living on their own, had good jobs (librarian, salesperson, tutor, university student), were dating, and had friends. One was even married. And this was in the days before any effective treatments were available! The first thing I learned is that the natural history of high-functioning autism includes remarkable improvement, even in the absence of intervention.

Fred's story was an illustration of one of the best outcomes I encountered. I arranged to meet him outside his apartment one evening. I arrived on time, which was unusual for me, keenly aware that many people with autism were quite rigid about their routine. For all I knew Fred had a specific schedule and would be very upset if I were late. Instead, nobody was there. I waited and waited, wondering where he might be. I was about to leave when a young man, dressed quite elegantly in suit and tie, arrived breathlessly and apologized for being late. Was this Fred, the person with autism I was supposed to meet? It was indeed. He explained that he had been tutoring a high school student in geography and that it had taken longer than expected. He asked politely whether I had eaten, and when I said that I had not, he suggested we go out to dinner. I was completely taken aback. He was so polite and even thoughtful about whether I was hungry. I would never have guessed that this young man was "autistic" given my recollection of the severity of his symptoms as a child. His medical chart described temper tantrums, rigid behavior, lack of social interaction with adults and other children, and intense resistance to change. Was this the same person?

We drove to the restaurant in my car. It was one of those small Italian neighborhood restaurants that served homemade pasta. We talked for a long time about his childhood, his current situation, and his aspirations for the future. He had very few memories of being autistic; in fact he could not remember anything prior to five years of age. He was in a class with other children with autism, which turned out to be an unpleasant experience. He had always been interested in maps; indeed, that was his obsession as a child. It was remarkable to me that geography was now his career, that he had been able to take an "obsession" and turn it into a useful vocation. He earned money as a tutor but was hoping for a more promising career in teaching. Anybody looking at us eating our pasta at the table would imagine we were talking about girls, sports, or the latest gossip at the office. Instead we were talking about being autistic, what that was like from the inside, and what was left of the disorder as part of his personality. He felt that the only residual impairment he experienced was anxiety in social situations. He had dated girls, intended to marry eventually, but felt a little anxious in group settings. He was animated, funny, made jokes about himself, used lots of gestures. Yes, he was a bit stiff and formal but hardly different from many people his age. Was Fred normal? How different was he from millions of others who grew up as typical children? His development was indeed a triumph. Admittedly, this type of outcome is quite rare, but it's not impossible. In my study, it occurred only in individuals with autism who were quite bright. What was so remarkable in Fred's case were the dreadful interventions he had received as a child, so I could not even begin to guess what had made a difference in his situation. One clue, though, was provided by the story of Hershel.

Hershel's outcome was perhaps not as spectacular as Fred's but was amazing in its own way. He lived with his mother in the suburbs and was enrolled at the local university. He was taking history and a few general liberal arts subjects, but he was barely passing and was receiving extra tutoring. I went to his home, a modest bungalow set among mature trees on a quiet street. It soon became clear to me that this was a deeply religious family. Hershel was a quiet young man and wore a yarmulke. He spoke little and answered my questions politely but succinctly. He lived an isolated life but attended synagogue regularly. He had some friends but saw them only through the synagogue. He had few hobbies or outside interests. He was unclear about his future but was very concerned about his marks at university. He was perhaps too concerned about graduating to the exclusion of all else. He did not see the degree as a means to an end but an end in itself.

Still I was astonished at how well he had done over the years. There was no possibility that the early diagnosis was wrong, as I discovered when I later reviewed the chart. Hershel had had many autistic symptoms as a child and was reported to have a fairly severe learning disability. That made his academic accomplishments all the more remarkable.

What I remember most vividly about the interview, however, was Hershel's mother. She was a forceful woman, though small in stature. We sat at the dining room table, surrounded by family photographs of children and relatives from the "old country." She talked vividly about those early years, the pain, the anxiety, and the worry about the future.

When she first noticed something was not quite right with Hershel, she took him to a specialist at a large teaching hospital. The specialist said the boy was autistic and the mother should make plans to have him schooled separately from other children and eventually institutionalized. Hershel's mother listened to all this with a stoic countenance, thanked the doctor for those words of advice, and then quickly dismissed everything he said. She looked at me sternly and said, "When I left that office, I swore I would make a mensch out of that boy if it was the last thing I did!"

After that clinical encounter, Hershel's mother enrolled her son in a regular kindergarten in his neighborhood school and signed him up for all the activities appropriate for a boy brought up in a religious home. She remembers fighting with all the professionals at the school board, the petty clerks in the recreation programs for children, the doctors who thought they knew better. Nobody could challenge her determination to help her son. He may have been ostracized, he may have been made fun of, but at the end, who could say how he would have turned out if she had not fought for him so valiantly and courageously? She had an indomitable will that few could withstand or resist. What she did was not fashionable in the Toronto of that era. There was no evidence then, as there is now, that mainstreaming children with autism was more beneficial in most circumstances than setting up special schools and segregating them from their peers. No doubt, the professionals in their offices, with their 2.5 children at home, nodded sagely at case conferences to each other and said that she was overinvolved, that she was in denial about her son's disability. But what perhaps few of these professionals realized was that it was this advocacy that had made much of the difference in Herschel's life.

Susan's life told a rather different story, triumphant in its own right in spite of the abject poverty in which she and her father lived. She resided in the heart of Toronto, in a rather run-down neighborhood. I remember standing on the porch of her house, ringing the doorbell. The house was in considerable disrepair, the paint was peeling, and the screens were coming off the windows. Eventually Susan came to the door. She looked at me quizzically and then remembered we had an appointment and invited me in. She had been upstairs, she told me, doing some calendrical calculations. She ushered me into a small living room. Calendars from different years were hung haphazardly on the walls, all showing the same month. An elderly, and obviously infirm, gentleman was sitting slumped in a chair, watching a game show on TV with the volume turned up very loud. I introduced myself politely, but I soon realized he was suffering from some type of hearing impairment. Susan told me her mother had died some years ago. She now looked after her father. They were visited occasionally by a social worker and some home help, but for the most part Susan did the shopping and cooking and cleaned up the house on a regular basis. She had no daytime employment, did not go to any sheltered workshops, but spent her time in her room poring over calendars and movie magazines. She was quite happy with her life and wished for little else.

Years ago, when her mother was alive, she got Susan into a routine of cooking and doing light housework. It had taken a long time, but again she must have been a forceful person, as eventually she was successful in teaching her daughter to look after herself and the house. Once that routine was established, it had a life of its own, and now that her mother was gone, the routine was all that allowed her to look after her father and still live at home. Her triumph was that in spite of her disability she managed to look after her father. One of the benefits of rigidity is that it makes a routine, once established, so much a part of a person with autism's life. She may not have considered looking after her father such a burden, but I could only wonder at her capacity to make a life out of these circumstances. It was the capacity for autistic routines that saved this family. Susan just went about her business quietly and efficiently, but I was aware of the enormous effort and training that had gone into the establishment of that routine in the first place. Her mother must have had that indomitable will I had seen so many times in other families.

*   *   *

I tried that day to give Melody and Sean something to hold on to, something to use as a touchstone as they navigated their future with Teddy. I hoped the things I had learned from these stories would illustrate the potential for goodness in people with autism and ASD and the traces of courage and fortitude found in the most unlikely places. I wanted to emphasize the common elements I found in those stories of children who had done well.

Perhaps those elements as well as other lessons learned from more recent outcome studies could illustrate how the children with ASD arrived at where they are, from where they were.

One common theme is that focusing on reducing the level of impairment and improving functioning seems to be more effective than trying to eliminate autistic symptoms alone. The first things to improve in young children with ASD are attending to instructions, simple language skills, compliance with simple commands, and later on skills of daily living such as dressing, eating at the table, going out into the community, and so on. These improvements show up in both treatment studies and those that describe outcome, independent of any particular treatment. Autistic symptoms, particularly those that reflect the social reciprocity impairment and restricted interest legs of the autistic triad (see Chapter 1), rarely disappear completely; they often became more subtle, more private, or more circumscribed to a specific time and place. It seems easier to improve IQ scores than autistic symptoms themselves. The autistic symptoms seem to decrease on their own as functional skills in communication, social interaction, and play improve. Working on these functional skills becomes an important avenue for further community inclusion in school, on soccer teams, in Scouts, and elsewhere, which in turn improves the child's daily living skills even more. It was certainly true that parents who advocated forcefully on their child's behalf to be included in these types of community activities and settings had done better in my outcome studies, as shown by the story of Hershel.

Another important lesson is that there is a false dichotomy between teaching the child a new skill to improve functioning and doing something to the environment to accommodate to those deficits. Most often, the environment includes people with whom the child interacts or the rules and regulations that govern their interactions in school or other community settings. The key is to get those people to readjust their expectations and to work around the limitations that having ASD imposes on the child. Changing the child cannot occur without changing the environment; a continuous dialogue occurs between those two poles. Once the environment (or people) accommodates to the child, it's easier to intervene with the child, which in turn changes people's attitudes to be more accepting of eccentricity.

I saw Sean and Melody some months later for a follow-up appointment. Teddy was now in a special day care, he was receiving speech therapy and help in playing with peers, and was enjoying going to school. Sean and Melody were much more relaxed about his situation and were willing to give this intensive approach a chance. They had come to appreciate small gains in his development and were very pleased with each new word that Teddy seemed to understand. A smile broke across Melody's face as she told me about her race with him through the kitchen to the living room and how Teddy looked at her one day in surprise and laughed at her silliness.

I know times of disappointment are inevitable for parents, that at the end of the day, the outcome for their child may not be as good as they had hoped for. But at least it is usually better than what they feared. It is important to be optimistic without being foolish. What is most essential is to persevere and to be determined to make sure that your child is included in any environment that is suitable, even if that environment has to be changed to accommodate the child. Quiet perseverance and determination are the advocacy skills that any parent needs, not to advocate for a cure—that is perhaps too much—but to advocate for understanding and acceptance. In that way, change and improvement occur over time. It may not come right away, but it will come.

The triumphs of a child with ASD during development are just as real and as impressive as the triumphs of any typical child. They are different but no less magnificent for all that. To see those triumphs is no easy matter. They are not obvious to the naked eye, particularly if one takes the perspective of typical development as a yardstick. But if one sees the world as the children with ASD do, if one takes the time to appreciate their perspective, then the triumphs and the successes become apparent and meaningful. It's not where a child ends up that counts; it's where he or she has come from that is the true measure of a child's courage and fortitude. Justin, Jeremy, Tom, and all the other adults with autism and ASD have the right to stand tall among their more typical peers. And Melody and Sean are coming to see that as well as Teddy grows up and gets better—and what more telling sign of that than when he laughs at his mother for being silly?

Chapter 8

Sally, Ann, and Danny

Accepting the Enigma,
Moving Beyond the Cause

I come down the stairs late, and slightly breathless, for my afternoon appointment. I am confronted by what looks like a day care class outside the office; three very young children, two girls and a boy, are running up and down the hall, shouting gleefully. They are watched rather anxiously by their parents, who in turn are watched rather anxiously by two grandparents. I quickly usher the entire family into my office. It's so crowded that there is little room for the children to run around. The noise level is deafening, but I try to gather some information, turning back and forth from the adults to the children, who are very beautiful, with wispy blond hair and penetrating blue eyes.

The parents tell me the children are triplets. The girls, Sally and Ann, are identical twins, and the boy, Danny, is a fraternal twin. The mother, Joan, used to be a shop assistant; she is dressed in white jeans and a sweater and wears glasses. She looks completely and utterly exhausted. The father, Dave, is a machinist who works the midnight shift. He has just woken up to drive everybody to the appointment. Both parents are very worried about the children's development and wonder whether they might have autism. They have no other children at home. They look at me anxiously as if I might give them an immediate and perhaps reassuring answer. Instead I gather some information to understand what might have happened and whether it is true that lightning has struck three times in the same family at the same instant.

The pregnancy itself was uneventful, although Joan experienced quite a bit of morning sickness. The triplets were born early by C-section amid much joy and celebration. All three weighed under four pounds. After the birth, the babies did well in the neonatal unit and were off the respirators in twenty-four hours. They were in the hospital for only nine weeks and then were sent home. There was quite a lot of fuss among the nursing staff, and everybody was amazed at how well the babies had done. When the family left the hospital, they were showered with presents and given a big send-off. Even the local community newspaper was there taking pictures. At home, the parents tried to cope with the demands of caring for triplets. Joan read everything she could about multiple births, searched the family tree for other twins born to relatives, and enlisted the help of her parents and friends at the earliest opportunity.

They had regular appointments with the family doctor and the pediatrician and followed all directions meticulously. Joan and Dave became concerned with the children's development at around eighteen months, when they noticed that their babbling was not progressing to speech. At their two-year appointment in the clinic the pediatrician wondered whether the triplets might have autism based on their social behavior and lack of interest in communicating. The parents were shocked and alarmed. The pediatrician asked whether I could see them as soon as possible.

*   *   *

The children wander around the room, picking up Lego pieces but not really playing with them. The boy sits quietly in his mother's lap, asking for nothing. One girl falls down accidentally but does not cry or go to her mother. The children approach their parents infrequently, and when they do, there is little response to parental communication. At age twenty-four months, only one of the girls is showing any communicative intent by bringing a plastic container to her parents and asking for help in opening it to see what's inside. The three children mill around us, largely oblivious to me and to their parents. Joan speaks their names, one by one, but they do not turn around to see who calls them.

Danny bumps into me as if I were not there, Sally lines up some action figures and babbles to herself, Ann is fascinated with the light on my power bar. There is little in the way of social interaction among the children and little desire to communicate either with me or with the parents or grandparents, who now include me in their anxious gaze. At home, the girls like to watch old Disney videos, *Fantasia* especially, and Barney. Danny loves to jump on the couch for hours on end.

At the conclusion of the interview the parents and grandparents want to know only two things: Do the triplets have ASD, and what possibly could have caused this tragedy? How is it possible that three children born into the same family and at the same time all have ASD? I tell them it is perhaps too early to tell, but we should do some assessments of communication and cognition, get them into day care, and follow them closely. I will see them again in three and then six months. I tell myself that it's likely they have autism, but I know that a diagnosis at twenty-four months of age can be difficult, especially in twins, who are often speech delayed, so I decide to wait a bit. In any case, they will receive useful interventions in day care, so there will be no real delay in receiving services.

*   *   *

Another couple, Ron and Carol, ask me to see their son, Robert, who is now ten years old. I saw him for the first time some six years ago for a diagnostic assessment, but the purpose of this current appointment is to discuss possible causes of his autism. They have two younger children, ages four and five, both of whom are doing very well, and there is no history of autism on either side of the family. Carol and Ron, who are both lawyers, have seen many physicians about their son's autism. I vividly remember the history from the first time I saw the family. Apparently Robert developed very nicely until age eighteen months. He had about fifty words, was always smiling, responsive, and engaging. All this could be seen from the videotape of his first birthday that his parents kindly supplied me. It showed him happy, blowing out the candles, clapping his hands, and laughing at all the goings-on. But a few weeks after his vaccination needle at eighteen months, he became quite ill. One night he developed a high fever and had a prolonged convulsion that terrified his mother. He turned blue and started shaking as she held him tenderly in her arms. Carol described this night as if it were yesterday—the layout of the bedrooms in the house, the cries that awoke her in the middle of the night, the frantic scramble to find the phone and call an ambulance. She was convinced he was going to die. Robert was rushed to the hospital, but thankfully he did not have any more seizures. A few weeks after he came home from the hospital, however, he seemed to be a different child. He became lethargic, withdrawn, and reclusive, and over the next few months he stopped using his words altogether. He no longer smiled or brought objects to show his parents. He was cranky and irritable. Soon he started to show a fascination with bits of paper, ripping them up into little pieces, rolling them into little balls, and throwing them down the stairs. He would also spend hours flipping through the pages of his father's law books.

His parents were of course devastated by this turn of events. They had in effect lost their son; to them it felt as if he had died that night of the convulsion. Robert's mother was deeply distressed, and his father tried to be supportive, but he too felt a deep loss. They started seeing doctors in their local area but became angry, frustrated, and disappointed with the answers and opinions they received.

Eventually, Robert was given a diagnosis of autism by a specialist. But this did not end his parents' search; they now began an intensive and exhaustive search for a cause. They were convinced that something must have caused this regression in his social and communication skills—perhaps the vaccination. But they could not get the doctors to agree with them. It's true that regression like this can occur in about thirty percent of children with autism, usually in the eighteen- to twenty-four-month range. In the vast majority of cases, though, no discernible cause can be identified, and this can cause the parents a great deal of frustration. (This is not the same as disintegrative disorder, another ASD subtype, where the period of normal development is much longer than twenty-four months.)

For this new appointment with me, Ron and Carol have sent along a rather large stack of medical documents that chronicles the story of these investigations and consultations carried out around the country. Robert had several magnetic resonance imaging (MRI) and computerized tomography (CT) scans done and many other investigations, but nothing specific showed up. Similarly, all the blood tests gave results in the normal range. In the meantime, he became very fussy about food and would eat only chicken nuggets and drink apple juice. He soon developed frequent diarrhea. As a result of this new set of problems, he had several gastrointestinal investigations, including X rays of his digestive system and biopsies of his intestines. These produced some nonspecific findings suggestive of colitis. Ron and Carol had read on the Internet recently that vaccinations for measles, mumps, and rubella (MMR) can cause colitis and that this may alter the permeability of the digestive system, allowing toxins into the bloodstream. According to this Website, these toxins affect the brain and can cause autism. Now Robert was on a gluten- and casein-free diet, which his mother found very difficult to implement and Robert refused to eat. As a result, dinner time was always difficult and a frequent setting for conflict.

Ron and Carol's journey around the country with Robert amounted to one long and arduous search for an answer. This vaccination–colitis–autism connection was the latest hypothesis they were pursuing. Ron and Carol felt strongly that pinpointing a cause would lead to more effective treatments. It would provide concrete evidence of pathology that would suggest a treatment intervention like a change in diet or other approaches such as the hormone secretin, allergy pills, and yeast infection pills—all interventions that have at one time been promoted as a "cure" for autism but that have little documentation of effectiveness. What was sad to see in the notes was that over the years there was little discussion of realistic, evidence-based treatment options for the autism that would improve Robert's functioning but that make no claims about "cure." There had been no behavioral interventions to improve his social skills, few attempts to teach him augmentative forms of communication, and little in the way of sustained opportunities for inclusion in regular school. Ron and Carol argued that since the autism came on suddenly in a child previously well, it must have been caused by something that, when removed, might cure the autism and give them back their son. This pursuit, though, prevented their taking up opportunities to lessen the degree of disability through the standard evidence-based interventions available.

It was a difficult interview. Robert sat patiently in his chair, showing little interest in the toys that were available, rocking back and forth, sitting on his hands. He did want to read some of the books on my shelves, which I was happy to share with him. But I made sure I gave him some old books that he could rip apart at will. He was still having difficulty communicating and only occasionally used single words to ask for food or books, but he was able to sing songs from children's shows. He spent all his time at home, was not involved in community activities like swimming lessons or other recreational activities. He ran around the house for hours on end when not watching TV. Not much had changed in the years since I had seen him last. The parents sat on either side of him and were grim faced, almost like battle-scarred victims of the health system. There was no cheerful greeting, no catching up on what had happened over the interim, no discussion about what was new in the field of autism.

"What we want to know is what tests can we do to see if the vaccination caused his autism?"

"I don't think there are any," I reply, knowing that this answer will not satisfy.

"What about urinary peptides or blood levels of proteins? Other research we have seen on the Net shows that kids with autism after the vaccination have abnormal levels of these chemicals."

"I would be interested in seeing those results. I find it hard to keep up with research that is only posted on various Websites. To me that could mean that the authors would prefer to not have their research scrutinized by members of the scientific community. That's usually the minimum requirement for accepting as valid what people might claim to be true."

"That's because most doctors don't want to believe the research."

I sighed. This was going to be a long interview.

*   *   *

I see Joan and Dave and the triplets six months later. They have now had several months of intervention in a community child care setting with lots of extra support from people knowledgeable about autism. If the impairments in the children were transient or caused by something other than autism, one might expect that there would be a large improvement. I learn that the triplets have adapted well, they enjoy going to day care, are eager to get ready for school, and quickly participate in the activities. They do not need time to warm up but are at the sensory bins first thing. Sally is using her few words more communicatively, but the other two are still not talking. The difficulties in social interaction remain, and the preference for repetitive and solitary activity is still very strong. They are not really interacting with the other children in day care; they still love to watch videos; and Danny still jumps on the couch for hours at a time. I tell the parents that I think the triplets do in fact have autism. They take all this in stride. A few tears well up in Joan's eyes, but she tells me she has already done her crying. Given the enormity of the predicament, I perhaps naively expected them to be more distraught, but of course they knew all along what was wrong with the children. Most parents are, in fact, devastated by the diagnosis and do their mourning in private, hopefully with the support of family and friends. It is parents who have trouble accepting the diagnosis, who do not mourn, who have the most difficult time moving on.

I ask Joan and Dave how they are handling the situation. They tell me that other people are worse off then they are—some children with autism are violent and aggressive, they tell me—and at least their kids are compliant and easy to handle. In some ways having three affected children is easier; one does not know any different. If you are prepared to deal with one child, you may as well be prepared to deal with others. Now that they know the diagnosis, they want to know how it is possible to have triplets with autism. Why is their family so special?

*   *   *

The search for a cause is a powerful drive for parents of children with ASD. One way we cope with tragedy is to try to find out why it befalls us. Parents will sometimes search relentlessly for a cause as it gives them a sense of control over the situation, but also perhaps because they have not fully accepted the diagnosis and all it entails. The general public has such a terrible image of autism that it makes acceptance hard. Most people in the community think of people with autism as violent, self-abusive, chronically dependent, and in need of institutionalizing in mental hospitals. Endlessly searching for a cause stems in part from a refusal to accept this picture, which is quite appropriate. But the diagnosis also entails an understanding of what we know about the causes of autism and what we consider to be evidence-based treatments. In some sense, not accepting the evidence base amounts to not accepting the diagnosis and all it entails. As mentioned in Chapter 7, this can be a real problem if it delays the start of effective early interventions. There is now good evidence that interventions that begin as early as possible can make a real difference to long-term outcomes; children with autism can improve, if not be cured. But it requires concerted effort and a determination to begin early and move on from trying to find a cause.

I tried to explain to both sets of parents the current understanding of the causes of autism. The explanation doesn't take long as we know so little and there are still large gaps in our knowledge. About ten percent of children with ASD have some other form of neurological disorder that disrupts the brain in a significant way. As a result, some children with diseases such as tuberous sclerosis or fragile-X syndrome also have autism as a secondary consequence of their neurological disability. Often such children are severely cognitively delayed with profound learning disability. In those cases, the autistic symptoms and behaviors are associated features rather than a primary concern. If a child is mute and has no play skills because of profound learning disability, the child may display behaviors also seen in higher-functioning children with autism. In these cases, the autistic features are a result of the severe cognitive disability, not necessarily a result of autism. Why some children with tuberous sclerosis develop autism and others do not is a mystery. In general, the more severe the cognitive disability, whatever the cause, the greater the likelihood that signs of autism will also be present, though this is not always the case.

Of the other ninety percent of cases of ASD without an accompanying neurological disorder we know even less, but certainly more than we used to. We know the disorder is inherited in some fashion; autism and ASD are genetic disorders, though what is inherited, and how, is still very much an open question. About three to five percent of the siblings of children with autism also have autism. Although this is a very low rate, it's much more common than in the general population (roughly two per thousand), suggesting that autism runs in families. But the best evidence for the genetic cause of autism comes from comparisons of twins, at least one of whom has autism. Several studies have compared the rates of autism in the co-twins of identical and fraternal twins. Twins share the same intrauterine environment but differ essentially in the number of genes they have in common. Identical twins share one hundred percent of their genes, whereas fraternal twins share, on average, fifty percent of their genes. The results of these twin studies are conclusive; the identical co-twins of autistic children have autism much more frequently than fraternal co-twins. This can be explained only by the action of genes that confer susceptibility to autism and ASD. The chance that non-twin siblings will have autism is three to five percent, much lower than the incidence in identical twins. This must be because multiple genes are involved in the etiology or some environmental factor interacts with genetic susceptibility. This does not mean that environmental factors are irrelevant; in fact there is good evidence that thalidomide and maternal anticonvulsants taken during pregnancy may cause autism. Other environmental risk factors may exist (but have not yet been discovered in spite of years of research), and if they do, they may exert their influence in the context of genetic vulnerability.

But the genetics of the disorder are complex. There are at least four findings that cannot be explained by our current understanding. First, not all identical co-twins are affected—usually about sixty percent (a finding similar to many other developmental and neurological disorders). If there were a simple genetic explanation, one might expect all identical co-twins also to be affected with autism. Second, the low rate of siblings who themselves are affected with autism/ASD and the sex ratio of more boys than girls make it unlikely that the disorder is caused by a single gene acting in isolation, like the gene for other disorders, such as cystic fibrosis and Huntington's disease. Multiple genes must be involved, but how they interact is completely unknown. Third, it's difficult to understand why the prevalence of the disorder is not decreasing. After all, the vast majority of people with autism do not have children; they do not pass their genes on to their offspring. If the disorder is genetic, it should be less common now than it was generations ago; the genes should be becoming less prevalent. In fact we know that people with autism were described at least three hundred years ago by Itard, who wrote about the wild boy of Aveyron. If anything, the number of children receiving the diagnosis has increased over the last ten years or so, but whether the disorder itself is more common, we simply do not know.

It's true that there has been a dramatic increase in the number of children receiving an ASD diagnosis in the last fifteen years or so. A lot of concern has been raised that the increase coincides with the widespread introduction of the MMR vaccine, and this has been one of the findings that has fueled the controversy about the vaccine. The most important point to remember is that there is no evidence that the disorder is actually increasing in the community; it's the number of children being recognized in the community that is increasing. There are no community surveys that have been done twice in the same area using the same measurement tools that could tell us definitively whether the increase is real, or an artifact of better recognition. In fact, we have reasons to believe that changes in recognition could account for a large part of the increase:

1. The diagnostic criteria for autism have been broadened to include a larger number of children.
2. The diagnosis can now be applied to more children at both ends of the spectrum (that is, those who are high functioning and those who are low functioning).
3. The diagnosis is now applied more often to children with other disorders such as Down syndrome and tuberous sclerosis.
4. We are now able to make the diagnosis more easily in very young children and adults.

The most striking data on the increase in prevalence come from the state of California, which keeps good records on children with developmental disabilities. California has reported a dramatic increase in the number of children with autism but also a dramatic *decrease* in children receiving a diagnosis of mental retardation (though to be fair, this finding has been challenged as well). It's certainly possible that children who in the past would have received a diagnosis of mental retardation are today receiving a diagnosis of ASD, especially since in many jurisdictions it's easier to get services with an autism diagnosis than with a mental retardation diagnosis.

Ron and Carol raised a fourth problem in our discussion. They rightly point out that no one else in their family has autism, no uncles or cousins. In their case the other children in the family are completely normal and there are no extended relatives with the diagnosis. How is this possible, if the disorder is inherited? I explained to them that, in fact, there are several inherited disorders where there is little family history (like breast cancer and senile dementia), even though some of the genes that cause these disorders have now been identified. In addition, other studies have shown that single autistic-like traits, that are not severe enough to warrant a formal diagnosis, are found more commonly among relatives of children with ASD than in the general population. Traits such as social isolation, intense interests and hobbies, rigidity, unusual ways of communicating, and perhaps learning problems are not uncommonly seen in relatives from both sides of the family; about twenty percent of relatives are affected with these traits. So, although autism may be very rare among extended family members, there is some evidence that individuals with unusual personalities are found in the family tree.

Now, it may be that once a diagnosis of autism is given, parents search their family tree and perhaps overidentify ASD-like traits in individuals that they might otherwise not recognize. People often look at their relatives with a new perspective and wonder if they might have a mild form of ASD. "It was from your side of the family." "No, it was from yours—just think of your cousin William!" parents will sometimes argue. On the other hand, these data may indicate that the genes for autism/ASD are not uncommon in isolation and that the full disorder occurs when certain genes combine or when genes interact with certain intrauterine environments.

So, no genes for autism have yet been identified, but several promising leads have turned up. Progress has been rapid in the last few years, but it's likely that many more years of work will be needed before we have a very clear picture of how these genetic factors cause autism/ASD.

* * *

Joan and Dave seem quite satisfied with the explanation. After all, as the parents of three affected children, the idea that autism is a genetic disorder seems quite obvious to them. But other parents like Ron and Carol are not so easily mollified, especially when the onset of autism is so closely connected with an event like a vaccination. To them the evidence that autism is caused by vaccinations is too compelling. There is even a new name for this condition, "new variant autism," another subtle indication perhaps of not accepting the diagnosis. I point out that, contrary to what they may have read, there is now good evidence that vaccinations do not cause colitis and that the measles virus (from the vaccine) has not been identified from biopsies of the intestines of children with autism. Moreover, it is not unusual for autism to appear at around eighteen months of age and, as mentioned earlier, about thirty percent of children with autism do have this history of a regression in social and communication skills. But this regression occurs just as often before as after their vaccination. Based on whole-population data, it seems that there is no clustering of the onset of autism around the time of vaccination and no decreased rate of autism in children who were not vaccinated with MMR. The events surrounding Robert's vaccination and the subsequent development of autism may have been a coincidence, or his brain might already have been vulnerable to experiencing a febrile convulsion, though the autism had not yet declared itself fully. I conclude by saying that the evidence does not suggest that vaccines and altered gut permeability play a role in causing autism. Ron and Carol, though, seem unconvinced.

It is at this point that as a clinician I run straight into the limits of science. I recognize that my explanation appears pathetically meager, that it provides so little solace to grieving parents. The story I can tell is so vague and abstract. There are so many gaping holes that it is unsettling. It gives people very little to hang on to. In the face of this mystery and the limits of what I can tell them about what caused their child's disorder, many parents quite understandably lose faith in the ability of science to tell them anything with certainty and turn to these alternative theories of cause instead. And they turn all the more readily to these alternatives when they also promise a cure.

There have been many alternative theories about the causes of autism. These include the idea that autism is caused by a fear of social interaction, with subsequent retreat from others, by a motor disorder that makes speech impossible, by a sensory abnormality that encourages withdrawal, by yeast infections, by allergies, by Lyme disease, by deprivation, and so on. The list goes on and on, and a new theory seems to crop up every two years or so. The attraction of many of these theories is that they suggest immediate cures such as (in order of the preceding "causes") holding therapy (hold the child tight to get through to him or her), facilitated communication (hold the child's hand while typing), auditory integration therapy (put headphones on the child and train him or her to hear other frequencies), antifungal medications, steroids, vitamins or secretin, or play and psychotherapy. Eventually every one has been discredited by good-quality scientific evidence or simply by the failure of the promised cures to materialize, in which case they just fade away.

The problem with these alternative theories is that there is always some evidence to support them, though the various bits and pieces cannot be brought together into a convincing story based on the evidence rather than on conjecture. For example, there is no question that children with ASD have allergies; it is just that the rate of allergies is no greater than in children without ASD. There is some evidence that children with autism may have depressed immune function; this may indeed make them more susceptible to colds and the flu and may be associated with an increased frequency of allergies in some complicated way. But that is still a long way from saying that allergies *caused* autism in the child. In fact, it may be that the immune system is depressed because the brain of the child is dysfunctional in a number of ways. The brain exerts a powerful influence on the immune system, so the cause-and-effect relationship may in fact be the opposite of what these explanations propose.

It is also true that blood levels of certain proteins may be unusually high or low among children with autism. Changing the diet of a child with autism may lead to changes in these levels of proteins. But it is quite another thing to say that these children have a leaky gut that has allowed these substances to enter the body and specifically to poison those brain systems or that the change in diet caused the improvement in behavior. That is pure conjecture. It is just as likely, if not more so, that the unusual food preferences and the restricted diet of children with ASD cause the abnormal levels of proteins in the blood and even the appearance of colitis in the gut. After a change of diet, the child may be better simply because he or she is handled in a different way, given more attention, a more structured daily routine, or because parents desperately want to see changes—any changes—rather than admit there was nothing they could do to help their child, a perfectly understandable motivation.

What these "scientific" proponents of the leaky gut and allergies have learned is to start with a few isolated findings and then weave a convincing story to tie these facts together into a hypothesis. But people too often mistake a hypothesis for a fact, and the distinction between evidence and conjecture is often blurred. The proponents of these alternative theories fill in the gaps in knowledge with educated guesses and don't consider other explanations that might conflict with their views. They use their authority as scientists or medical doctors to give their stories credence. The stories are good ones, on the surface they are logically coherent, and they have a beginning, a middle, and an end. That's why they are so attractive: The experts speak with authority, they don't admit to any shortcomings, and each problem has a ready answer. It's just that all too often the evidence is simply not there to back up the guesses. It may be an overstatement, but perhaps parents should mistrust any source of information that sounds too authoritative or claims to know the answers about autism.

A model postulating a simple cause and a simple effect makes for a convincing story. But the complexity of much of human diseases can no longer be captured by such simple models. With complexity comes ambiguity and uncertainty in the minds of parents. Into this state of mind, stories told by authorities (with little evidence to back them up) come creeping in and look more and more attractive. In contrast, the current understanding of what causes autism is so unsatisfying; the gaps in knowledge are not filled with guesses, but are left open for further discovery. Part of the difficulty for parents in coming to terms with autism is coming to terms with this ambiguity and uncertainty, tolerating it and going on. It's all part of the process of accepting the diagnosis and moving on to finding treatments that are reputable and have been supported empirically by well-conducted studies. There are treatments that work; they have been published in respected journals, and parents can use them—see the Resources section for sources of more information. Accepting the diagnosis, the ambiguity about cause, and the fact that treatments cannot cure autism but can improve function and quality of life makes it possible, and imperative, to move on.

The problem is that the distinction between junk science, or "pseudo-science" (or even worse, movie-of-the-week science), and evidence-based science is often subtle, arising as it does out of the dual nature of scientific activity. At first the scientist conducts an experiment or sets out to collect information by reducing complex systems into simpler ones. The scientific method is essentially a reductionistic attempt to collect evidence that is as free of bias as possible. In a good experiment, similar results are found by other scientists doing similar work with similar populations and instruments. The more the evidence from one investigation fits in with other pieces of evidence and with other discourses, the more true it is. But the scientist recognizes that the reduction to simpler models leads inevitably to error. Error is an essential part of the world and can never be eliminated entirely. That is why certainty is never possible. The second activity is just as important and consists of *interpreting* those facts or findings. The disparate findings have to be brought together into a story that makes sense in terms of what we already know. Scientists build models of the biological systems under investigation. These models are undeniably situated in a particular context, embedded in a particular culture and language. That context will inevitably influence how the story is told. It's impossible to understand the world outside of language. The essential difference between evidence-based science and junk science is the balance between empirical findings and interpretation. Simply put, junk science is more interpretation and storytelling than the evidence warrants. When the story involves a medical doctor valiantly trying to persuade the military–industrial–medical complex that the cure for autism is around the corner if only people would listen and wouldn't let their vested interests interfere, then the story becomes movie-of-the-week science.

But lest we become too self-satisfied with accepted forms of wisdom and reject dismissively and arrogantly these alternative theories, it's important to remind ourselves that the first theory of autism espoused by the medical establishment was that parents cause autism in their children. In his original paper, Kanner noted that the parents of the eleven children he described very often showed somewhat unusual behavior themselves; they could be obsessive, aloof, hard driving, or artistic, or had poor social skills. It's interesting to note that many of these individuals were psychiatrists or psychologists, though Kanner, who was otherwise so astute, missed the connection between occupation and unusual, rigid personalities! Kanner wondered whether the similarity in social impairment reflected a genetic contribution to the disorder, a very perceptive observation. At that point in American medicine, however, the field of child psychiatry was dominated by the psychoanalytic orientation, so this observation of clinical similarity between parent and child was interpreted to imply that the social impairments in the parents, particularly the mother, caused the same social impairments in the child. In other words, the disorder was caused by impaired mother–infant bonding. At one point Kanner appeared to share this view, but he quickly repudiated it and returned to a more biological explanation. However, the die had been cast, and several hundred papers were written on how mothers cause autism by ignoring their children and treating them badly. The term "autism" fell into disfavor and the term "childhood psychosis" was used instead to reflect this orientation. The possibility that the original observation could be more parsimoniously explained by genetic factors was overlooked. Children with autism were subjected to psychotherapy, and the parents were taken into treatment and encouraged to explore their feelings of aggression toward their child. Special schools were set up, most notably by Bruno Bettelheim in Chicago, who coined the phrase "refrigerator mother." He was later found to have falsified his qualifications when coming to the United States and was accused of abuse by some of the children resident at his school. Not surprisingly, the disorder was found very difficult to treat given these methods.

In the late 1960s and '70s the tide began to turn against this view. Scientists from outside the psychoanalytic camp began to report that children with autism were more often male than female, frequently had epilepsy, often suffered from profound developmental delay, had so-called "soft neurological signs," electroencephalogram (EEG) abnormalities, and were the children of perfectly normal parents, not some pair of cold fish. None of these findings could be accounted for by the refrigerator mother model of autism. By the mid-'70s, autism was seen finally as a disorder of brain development by most credible authorities. It had taken thirty years, but the science of child psychiatry moved slowly in those days! Now it is hard to keep up with the ever-expanding literature on the biology of ASD.

It is very instructive to read these early theories about what causes autism in light of what we know today. What is most striking is the certainty with which the experts spoke. They knew what caused the disorder. The possibility of error was never considered. Even though today we have a better understanding of what causes autism, we are also acutely aware of the limits of our knowledge, the possibility and inevitability of error, and the effect of context and history on interpretation. But the historicity of scientific interpretation does not render scientific truth meaningless.

Parents often are confused by this conflict of interpretations—genetics on the one hand and the leaky gut on the other. If the theory we believed in the past (that parents can cause autism) is untrue, what confidence can parents have in what scientists say today? How can they tell the difference between evidence and junk science when there is so much conflicting information on the Web, at conferences, in newsletters, in the media, and by word of mouth? The key is in the language. Skepticism is the heart and soul of good science. The language of good science is iconoclastic, argumentative, and critical. Nothing is accepted as true unless all the findings are accounted for and the interpretation is true to the evidence. The story must cohere with other discourses and narratives. As such it is a never-ending story; the whole story can never be told, because every new finding goes deeper and deeper into the heart of the matter. The British author Jeanette Winterson writes that the truth is precisely what we do not know—all truths are partial truths. In science, as in life, the more we know, the less we understand, or, perhaps more accurately, the closer we come to the mystery of things. The source of the mystery recedes farther and farther from our grasp as we approach it. It is like going up a river: Seeing one bend in the river only makes one aware of the next bend around the corner.

The problem is that good science is hard to access for most parents. It's published in high-impact journals, and the language is often technical, full of jargon, and not easy to digest. Publications are often communications between scientists and are not meant to be read by parents. That's unfortunate, and there must be a way for parents to obtain the most up-to-date evidence-based information. The World Wide Web is certainly accessible to many, but there is so much junk science on it that parents are all too often led astray. At the very least, parents should avoid all Websites that solicit business, whether it is clients for class action suits, consultations to help their children, medications, or any other product. Probably the best place to start are government Websites that have health information or public health libraries on the Web. These will also have links to other sites such as parent support groups or other sources of reputable information.

As a clinician answering questions about what causes ASD, I am very much aware of the enormous gulf between my aspirations to tell as complete and true a story as possible and the limitations of our methods to unravel these mysteries. For parents, this gulf is painful to experience and to tolerate. It can sometimes drive parents to years of fruitless exploration. The temptation to weave a convincing story to help parents understand their tragedy is strong. After all, parents have come to the expert for an informed opinion. I recognize this is a powerful encounter, and I am keen not to disappoint them. I am painfully aware of the limits of science, but I try not to transfer that anxiety to parents and not to pull any junk science out of the hat at the last moment to make them feel better. Part of the necessary therapeutic alliance is trust and respect. As the doctor who makes the diagnosis I am supposed know what I'm talking about. But the story I have to tell does not have an overall narrative, a grand and logical structure. It's a pastiche, a collage of isolated bits of information. It is a truncated narrative; not all the pieces fit together. Each part of the story is told from one particular perspective, and to be faithful to the science, disparate narratives need to be brought together. But the overall story is unsatisfying at the end. Ultimately it does not cohere. It's like a modern novel, difficult to read.

The allergists and leaky gut doctors and scientists have no such qualms. They cheerfully ignore the abyss between evidence and interpretation in their stories and plow ahead, writing stories that cohere, filling in the gaps with suppositions and guesses, confident that what they are saying can accommodate any intrusion of evidence. They glide over these gaps with facility. I envy their brazen confidence. I envy their ability to communicate a story that makes sense.

Good science is located at the holes in knowledge. It lives in the spaces between findings and stories. It explores them, lives in them, and celebrates them. It is the disjunction that fascinates the good scientist and distinguishes him or her from the junk scientist. The writer Annie Dillard says that the scientist is like the tightrope walker, who must never look down for fear of becoming aware of the emptiness of the foundation—the lure of simple explanations, the impact of the method on the findings, of the context on the interpretation of results. The point is that not all interpretations are equal, not all stories are the same, not all evidence is of equal value. There are rules of evidence. We can tell good science from junk science once we realize that good science is not the search for truth but an attempt to learn the error of our ways.

*   *   *

In the end there is no rational explanation for the cause of ASD, at least not now. The genetic evidence that I alluded to earlier refers to what we know about the *population* of children with autism and ASD. Such theories say little about Sally, Ann, and Danny. It is about *Robert* that Ron and Carol want answers, not some abstract notion of "children with autism," and I have so little to give.

The parents of these children are innocent victims of their genetic background. The possibility of giving birth to a child with autism is the sword of Damocles they carried over their heads from childhood. These autistic susceptibility genes are nobody's fault, but they are passed down from one generation to the next. Misfortune lies in wait for years, through our childhood, adolescence, and young adulthood. It causes grievous harm only when two people come together and create a new human being, usually a joyous and wonderful act. But misfortune and tragedy lie in wait. For these parents, their destiny is truly in their genes.

This tragedy is senseless and lies just the other side of our daily lives. It happens to innocent people—a shop assistant and a factory worker, two lawyers. What have they done wrong? Is it a test? Is it a punishment for some earlier mishap or error? In the face of misfortune, we reason like children and personalize the accident as somehow caused by us. These births force us to confront the enormity of our biology. For these families, their genes are their masters to some extent because the genes determine a life history for them. The search for causes leads ultimately to the incomprehensibility of misfortune and tragedy. But this is not like a Greek tragedy, where the hero has committed a crime against the gods and must be punished. The misfortune is senseless, and to that extent evil lurks in our genes. We are all fallible, all prey to biological mishaps, potentially denied the joy of hearing a child's voice in the house.

Having three affected children makes it easier for Joan and Dave to accept that the disorder is genetic than it is for Ron and Carol. The enormity of the evidence is so overwhelming. This has allowed them to move on to treatment and to caring for these children while at the same time trying to create some semblance of normal family life. The relentless search undertaken by Ron and Carol for a cause has made it difficult for Robert to be fully involved in a comprehensive treatment program. All families with a child with ASD must live with the ambiguity of never knowing the exact cause of their child's handicap. Ron and Carol may continue to search for something concrete, hoping that would give them a key to unlocking the mystery of treatment. The difficulty is that there is no definite answer, so this search has the potential to go on forever without a successful resolution. For some families, continuing to search is a way of not accepting the diagnosis of autism. All answers are ambiguous, and this ambiguity is very hard to live with. But the ambiguity has to be experienced and tolerated. Only then can parents move on to mourning for the "lost child" and then searching for an evidence-based treatment program.

Understanding that autism is caused by multiple genes that affect the development of the social brain does have implications for these evidence-based treatments, even if the connection may seem far-fetched at present. Because multiple genes are involved, interventions should target several developmental domains and include both biological and psychosocial methods. People often think that if a condition is caused by genes, it must be fixed and therefore can't be open to interventions. That is simply not true. First, there are many genetic disorders that are eminently treatable and can even be cured. Second, interventions can be targeted to the gene products causing the problems, or the diet can be supplemented to make up for the genetic defect (think of phenyl-ketonuria). Third, genes turn on and off during development. It is not inconceivable that once some of the genes that cause autism are discovered it may be possible to turn the gene off (if it is producing some abnormal protein) or on (if it is not functioning for some reason). Discovering the genetic causes of autism opens up the real possibility of finding biomedical interventions aimed at the underlying causes of the disorder that have more specific and long-lasting effects than the medications we currently have available.

Chapter 9

Trevor
Mobiles and "Miracles"

"*I*t's the strangest thing. He could stay in his crib for hours staring at that mobile. It just hangs there, suspended over the crib—bits of colored cardboard strung together with fishing line. I put it up there one day just for fun, and now he looks at nothing else. What could be so interesting about fishing line?"

Strange indeed for a toddler now three years old. Alice was a single mother who worked as a pediatric nurse at our local children's hospital. She had a pretty good idea of what normal child development looks like. She was here today to tell me about her son, Trevor. I knew Alice from her work at the hospital and agreed to see Trevor because she was worried he had autism.

"We just had a birthday party for him last week. I invited his grandparents and some kids from the street. He doesn't know any of them, but I felt I just had to, to see what his response would be. Well, he ignored everybody, even his grandparents. He just stared at the candles on the birthday cake, and once he finished opening up his presents, he fled to his room. I followed him up there and found him staring at that damn mobile. I was so upset I cried. I had to amuse those other kids till their moms came to pick them up. I have never been so embarrassed in my life. What a nightmare that was."

Trevor was lining up the Lego pieces across the table. He had curly blond hair and was dressed in blue overalls with a bulky sweater underneath. It was a cold and wintry day outside, and they had struggled to come to the appointment through a snowstorm. I wanted to make the trip as worthwhile as possible. I tried to move one of the Lego pieces, but Trevor cried out in protest. I tried to stack them, and he cried out even louder. I was concerned that he didn't want to play with me. I decided to quit while I was ahead.

"Why don't you try to play with the Lego pieces with him?" I said to Alice, thinking it would be easier to assess his social play with his mother than with a stranger.

She had noticed my chagrin. "It won't make any difference," she said. "He will cry with me too. If I pick him up to comfort him, all he does is cry. The only way I can soothe him is to place him in the crib and let him stare at that silly mobile."

It was that awful moment when I realized that she knew, and she realized that I knew, but we couldn't say anything to each other.

"How does Trevor communicate with you?" I asked.

"He pulls me by the hand, puts my hand on the fridge or on the crib if he wants to be put in there. He refuses to sleep in a bed by the way. Every time I try he gets incredibly upset and runs around the house looking for his crib. He doesn't use words yet. In fact, I first wondered whether he was deaf. When he lies in the crib and I call his name, he doesn't even turn around and look at me. He's so absorbed in those silly cardboard pieces that hang above him. Yet when I call his name and he's in the living room, he will turn without a problem. He can't be deaf."

We went through the rest of the developmental history and scheduled another time for me to do a structured play assessment with Trevor. This was an opportunity to press for social and communication skills using a set of toys that elicit communication acts from the child. He came in a couple of weeks later, and his mother and I managed to do some activities with him. It was clear that Trevor was not displaying age-appropriate social and communications skills. For example, I enjoy blowing bubbles with the kids and it is a useful tool for assessing social–communication skills. When I blow bubbles, a typical child will smile, look at me, look at his or her mom, express pleasure using words or sounds, and ask for more after bursting all the bubbles. Trevor did none of these; he just stood there waiting for me to send the next train of bubbles floating through the air. I also have a remote-controlled car that is very neat. I hide it behind some boxes in the room and set it going while the child is absorbed in some other activity. I called out Trevor's name while he was playing with the Lego and said "Look" while my gaze was directed at the car going round and round in circles. Trevor looked at neither me nor the toy. I then gave him the remote control. A typical child will proudly show his parents how he can make the car move and might even offer to share the device with them. Unfortunately, Trevor displayed none of these social–communication skills. The diagnosis was obvious, and I delivered the bad news.

Alice had been present many times when bad news had been delivered to other parents on the ward, and so she was quite prepared to hear it. "OK, so what do we do now?" Alice was eager to start working with her son on his social and communication skills as soon as possible. "I want to have a closer relationship with him. I want him to get better. I don't want him to be shunted aside as he grows up. He is my only child. I'm prepared to do anything."

I tried to reassure her that if we could get him into a treatment program soon, it would make a big difference to his development. There now was some persuasive research on early intervention and the difference it can make in improving outcomes. But the first step was to identify his treatment needs more specifically and for Alice to learn more about the various treatment options that were available. This takes some time. She turned to our treatment team to help her through this next phase. Alice went to information nights we ran at the hospital on treatment, joined the local parent support group, talked to team members about situations at home and to other parents who had older children. She read many different books on treatment, including the testimonials of miraculous recovery "if only one followed this or that treatment program." She also read the more sober textbooks and treatment manuals that provided a more balanced account. Then she went on the Internet and read about other treatment options that were less well known, that had not been scientifically evaluated but had received a lot of press and testimonial evidence of success.

But at the end of all this information gathering, she felt no farther ahead. Worse, she was beginning to feel frantic. She did not know where to start—so many options, so many choices to make. Alice found all this information bewildering and disorienting. She was terrified that if she made the wrong choice, or delayed treatment any longer, all hope for Trevor's progress would be lost. Some of the information she read applied to Trevor, but certainly not all of it did. Some interventions she could implement at home, but others were not appropriate either because Trevor already had some basic skills or else Alice did not have the resources or the time to implement the more time-demanding strategies. Yet she felt guilty because she couldn't do all the things that seemed to promise remarkable success if only she started right now. She just did not know where to begin. She told me she felt like she was in a dream, wandering around lost in some nightmarish carnival with all those flashing lights and "hucksters" yelling at her to try this ride or that game and promising instant riches. Like many parents, Alice found it impossible to sort through all the information and to decide what to use and what to discard.

This frantic search for the right treatment program is all too common. Parents are desperate to find solutions and become easily overwhelmed with information overload. The problem is that the information that is out there for parents is filled with specifics of this or that approach, without first explaining some principles, providing a framework to understand. In addition, much of the information that is out there is not scientifically valid, or evidence-based. Alice had gone off to read the treatment manuals in her haste to help Trevor without first developing a good understanding of ASD as a disorder—what its manifestations are, what the underlying deficits might be, what strengths can be exploited in the various treatment programs. Parents need that framework in order to evaluate the evidence for each treatment option. Understanding the inner world of the child with ASD and the struggles that parents must endure is part of the "art" of implementing treatment programs in real community settings and of sifting through the literature. Indeed this understanding is a prerequisite to beginning any form of treatment, especially early intervention, since it provides a framework for understanding the goals of therapy and where to begin, and suggests methods for achieving that end. The early intervention manuals have a lot of useful information on how to *do* things, but it's also important to understand context, which in this instance is the inner world of the child with ASD, so mysterious yet so familiar at the same time. Taking a little time to see how ASD is a manifestation of deficits in theory of mind, in weak central coherence, in executive function, and in visual attention is an important first step.

The first thing we needed to do for Alice was to help her enter Trevor's world at his own level. Alice needed to understand what went on in Trevor's mind, how he saw the world and experienced all its vicissitudes of change and challenge, the constant swarm of sensations and chaos and the patterns seen in the most unlikely places. Over time, Alice watched Trevor very closely, especially in his play activities and how he spent his time. She also watched him in his play group at the library, where she took him once a week to interact with other children. She talked to team members about the meaning of certain behaviors. She learned that Trevor had a different set of priorities, a different set of values from the rest of us. Trevor did not choose these values of his own free will; they were imposed on him by the contingency of his biology. Trevor's priorities were sensory—visual patterns and textures—not social interaction. His mother could see that he had an incredible memory for details; it was this that consistently caught his attention, not the presence of another person. From her work in the maternity unit in the hospital, Alice knew that babies were attracted by the human face. Trevor seemed to ignore faces but stared for hours at the mobile swinging over his crib. Alice also knew that toddlers were aware of where their mothers were at all times. Trevor, on the other hand, could watch cartoons all day long and never checked to see if she was still in the kitchen cooking dinner. Trevor's world revolved around a different axis, just as Heather's did (see Chapter 2)—it was as simple and yet as mysterious as that.

By observing her son closely in this way, Alice could now see how the fundamental deficits and strengths that affect all children with ASDs take shape in the autistic behavior of an individual child: How Trevor might ignore faces because he had no intuitive understanding of how facial expressions were a window into someone's thoughts and feelings. How the mobile was not a bunch of "silly cardboard pieces" to Trevor but an object through which Trevor saw facets of the intimate architecture of the world that most of us never notice. How communication, such a natural, automatic developmental achievement for typical children, was to her son as formidable an achievement as learning calculus at age thirty-six months. How frustrating it must be for Trevor to lack the skills of asking for help if he wants more bubbles blown his way, if he wants more juice. Alice began to imagine as well how important the ability to be soothed and comforted was for children. Children get bumps and bruises all the time; they get scared, feel lonely, feel hurt. Alice was sure that Trevor felt all these things too, but he would not come to her for comfort, and if she picked him up to soothe him, it had no impact. In fact, it must feel to him like he is in a vise grip. The world must seem a frightening and bewildering place for Trevor, and he had to face all these challenges alone.

With this understanding it now became possible to build a more positive relationship between mother and son. Alice learned to read Trevor's behavior as a communication of his internal state. She became more sensitive to the subtlest forms of nonverbal communication. Certain sounds meant that Trevor was unhappy; rocking was an indication of mounting anxiety about some anticipated change in routine. All of a sudden, Alice understood that Trevor was communicating all the time! It was just that he was using a different communication system. Alice's role was to break the code, and once she understood this, she became more patient, less likely to become angry and misinterpret Trevor's actions as willful and stubborn rather than as directed at keeping his world in order.

Alice and Trevor were now ready to begin treatment. She was getting a little frustrated with me because I kept postponing this discussion about treatment until she could integrate all the information about ASD and see how it applied to Trevor. But it is so important to stop the frantic search for a cure and understand the context of what having an ASD means to the child.

"When are we going to begin treatment, and what treatment are we going to use?" she kept asking me. I didn't mean to appear secretive, but there was a lot of information to impart about treatment, and that takes time. Spending a few months on assessment, understanding treatment needs, having a good appreciation of cognitive strengths and weaknesses is essential. Understanding the capacity for learning very simple skills takes time and is essential in ensuring that the treatment is delivered in as efficient and effective a manner as possible. Taking that time does not delay the initiation of treatment; in fact it is an essential part of treatment. Starting treatment too early can be delaying treatment as well if it leads to false starts.

There has been an important shift in the philosophy of treating children with autism and AS over the last decade. Part of the reason for that shift has been a greater awareness of what is realistic to expect in terms of treatment response and a greater appreciation of the unique features of ASD as a disorder that affects all aspects of development. In the past, the emphasis was on reducing autistic behaviors such as echolalia (repeating phrases), behavior problems, and motor mannerisms (such as rocking, spinning toys, finger flicking) using a number of techniques, including punishment. Some of the therapists who used such techniques also made extravagant claims of "cure" in the absence of well-documented changes in day-to-day functioning. The goal is now not so much to reduce or eliminate "autistic behavior" but rather to facilitate social and communicative competence and so reduce the degree of impairment in day-to-day functioning. In this way, the so-called autistic behaviors—the echolalia, the motor mannerisms, and the behavior problems—often diminish on their own. Reducing autistic behaviors should be a goal only if they interfere with daily functioning or with delivering therapy. In addition, punishments are no longer used. Not only are punishments unethical, but if one of the goals of therapy is to encourage the child to interact with others, particularly adults, then delivering punishments will only teach children with ASD to be wary of adults. Nor is it realistic to expect a cure, in spite of the claims of some testimonials. Sometimes, however, the degree of improvement can be quite remarkable and heartening.

This realization has been accompanied by increasing evidence that early intervention can make a significant difference to the growth and development of children with ASD. Children who are initially nonverbal can begin to speak, children who do not follow simple directions can now do so, children who are socially isolated can now start to play with other children. Problems remain in the core difficulties of theory of mind, of weak central coherence and executive function, but they seem less severe. The impact of treatment is such that children with autism look more and more like children with AS or atypical autism, and these latter two groups look more and more like children with learning disabilities or with attention deficit. They may not look or behave normally all the time, but they are on a more developmentally appropriate pathway.

The main approach to early intervention based on the available scientific evidence is "applied behavioral analysis" (ABA), combined with a developmental approach to autism. This generic method focuses on understanding the function that behavior plays in a particular situation and attempts to teach more developmentally appropriate behaviors with a well-defined set of learning methodologies. By integrating ABA with a developmental approach these skills are taught in a sequence that attempts to follow typical developmental processes. These integrated methods also take into account how children with ASD learn—how they process information, especially information with a strong social and communication component, at different stages of their development. This can be much more difficult to accomplish than teaching compliance or the utterance of simple words to indicate preference, and it's what makes the application of ABA to children with ASD more complicated than to children with more general developmental delays.

There are several forms of early intervention, but the two most well known are "discrete trial training" and naturalistic teaching or "social–

communication therapy." These are not mutually exclusive and can be seen as lying on a continuum from highly structured behavioral ABA approaches such as discrete trial training to more naturalistic "developmental" ones. Both ends of the continuum have been evaluated systematically and scientifically in a number of studies and have been found to be effective, though many unanswered questions remain. There are several different variations to each, but the two main therapies have much in common. They are both intensive, start early, involve twenty to forty hours of treatment a week, though admittedly administering more than twenty-five hours per week is very difficult in most circumstances. Both also employ behavioral strategies to facilitate learning. They are also intrusive to the extent that the child is not allowed to disengage from the world entirely and to retreat into repetitive and solitary play. Staff who deliver the treatment are highly trained, and parents are actively involved in setting goals and in administering the treatment program, and are also taught a number of techniques to foster social interaction, language, and play. Both include systematic attempts to generalize treatment gains from one setting to another. For example, if a child with autism learns to play with a therapist, there is no guarantee that he will be able to play with parents or siblings. These skills need to be generalized across people but also across settings (like from school to home). Both approaches emphasize understanding what function a certain behavior serves, how new skills can be established step by step, how to use rewards to reinforce more developmentally appropriate behavior, how to use structure and a visual schedule to make transitions easier, and how maladaptive behaviors can be eliminated.

But there are also some important differences. Discrete trial training concentrates on promoting compliance and simple cognitive, language, and attentional skills through a strict application of learning principles. Therapeutic sessions are highly structured and directive, are largely done one on one with an adult, and have a strong training component. An example of a session using discrete trial training might involve a child sitting behind a table with the therapist sitting opposite to remove any distractions. The therapist puts two pictures down on the table and asks the child to indicate whether these are the "same" or "different." If the child is correct, he is rewarded. If not, the trial is given again. This procedure is done over and over again till the child can indicate the correct answer several times in a row. Once that skill is mastered, the child and therapist go on to the next skill in the curriculum. That next skill tends to be a bit more developmentally advanced, but the procedure is the same. Eventually these component skills are put together, and the child now has to group pictures together that tell a story in a logical sequence. That helps sequencing in general, an important basic skill in learning to use language.

This strategy is ideally suited for children with autism but has never been evaluated on children with AS. Indeed, young children with AS seem more suited for a treatment program that focuses on social skills and on attempts to promote a wider range of interests. This second approach is more naturalistic and involves promoting social and communication skills in general by targeting the key deficits of children with ASD. The focus here is on basic social skills in eye contact, sharing an activity with an adult or another child, indicating wants and needs with respect to food or snacks, indicating pleasure in response to an adult activity such as tickling or singing a song. Interactions are often initiated by the child rather than by an adult; the adult tries to synchronize his or her responses to the child's behavior. These interventions usually start at home or with an adult therapist too but soon move into community settings such as school or day care, with appropriate professional and clinical supports. By encouraging children with ASD to be in such settings, the opportunity to learn more appropriate social and communication skills from other children is also enhanced.

The idea is that children with ASD have excellent visual learning skills. But instead of using these skills to mimic TV characters or Disney videos, they might use them to learn from other children. The teacher or therapist sets up situations that encourage or facilitate social interaction and communication between the child with ASD and a typical child. For example, a child with ASD may learn to take turns in a favorite game with a therapist. Then, once that is mastered, the therapist may introduce another typical child so that the three of them take turns. Then the therapist backs off and provides support for the child with ASD to play with the typical child and intervenes only when necessary. However, sometimes the behavior of the child with ASD is just too challenging to begin in this fashion, and some children need some form of discrete trial training to begin. Working on attention span, compliance, and understanding simple language can make it much easier to implement these more "naturalistic" interventions.

Both of these forms of ABA have been shown to be effective compared to doing nothing. However, we do not know which type of ABA is more effective and efficient—that is, gives the most gain for the least cost—because the different forms have never been compared directly.

Neither do we know how to combine them most effectively into one program, nor what type of intervention works best for what type of child with ASD. There are no evidence-based principles by which to choose interventions, and these types of treatment decisions are best made through educated guesses by both parents and professionals based on the individual characteristics of the child, the particular situation and context of the child, and the child's response to the intervention (hence the need for an extended assessment time). Trial and error is often warranted: "If it works, go with it!"

For some time, the therapeutic claims for discrete trial training were exaggerated in the popular press and by some professionals given the quality of the evidence so far published. The possible gains are now understood to be more modest but are still clinically important. In fact, the gains for children with autism who also have severe learning disability are limited. The approach seems to work best with children who have at least moderate degrees of learning disability. Social–communication therapies may be just as effective, cost much less, and be more naturalistic for some higher-functioning children who are able to benefit from this form of intervention. Many experts feel this is the preferred treatment for children with AS and even for children with high-functioning autism who are verbal. The problem is that not all children with autism or PDDNOS have the attentional, social, and communication skills to make the best use of naturalistic settings. In these circumstances it may be best to start with a program of discrete trial training and then move on to more naturalistic and incidental teaching when the prerequisite skills appear or alternatively to work on both approaches simultaneously. Identifying essential skills needed for social interaction, teaching them using discrete trial training, and then moving on to the social–communication therapies is a useful strategy adopted by many professionals who like to take the best of both approaches and combine them.

*   *   *

Because Trevor had a moderate degree of learning disability based on cognitive testing and was just starting to communicate with pointing and pulling, we decided to start working on some other pivotal skills using discrete trial training. Attending is an important prerequisite skill for many other social, communication, and play skills. We taught Trevor to come sit, look at an object, and look at the therapist in response to having his name called. Each time he did the correct action, he was rewarded with a paper star that he could add to his mobile. We also started with trials teaching him how to imitate actions with objects and sounds. Then we progressed to imitation of mouth movements, hand movements (touch your head, touch your elbow), then verbal imitation (imitate vowel sounds, sounds of letters, etc.). We also worked on understanding language using discrete trials to help him identify pictures, objects, and colors and then to discriminate between objects (point to the door when presented with a picture of a room). Then we got him to follow one- and two-step commands and to find hidden objects. We also designed a program to work on expressive language by presenting him with two objects and asking him to label which one he preferred. Once each skill was mastered, attempts were put in place to teach him the same skill with his mother, his main teacher at day care, and finally one of the other teachers with whom he was less familiar.

He now had some basic attention and compliance skills that would allow him to benefit from more formal and structured attempts to facilitate social and communication skills in the context of other typical children. We also set up some guidelines for parenting and interaction that were different from the way Alice usually interacted with him. First we placed him in a community day care setting, and the school hired a teaching assistant to work with him on a curriculum we provided based on an assessment of his social, communication, and play skills. We helped to set out a routine for his day so that it was highly structured with play time at home with his mother included so that she could work with him as well. With Trevor, Alice was taught to be intrusive and take every opportunity to interact with him. She would hide things or put them out of reach so that Trevor would have to come to his mother and ask for them. Alice would set aside some time each day to play with Trevor, to build things with his Lego pieces, do puzzles with him. She would consistently and enthusiastically reward all attempts at communication and social interaction or attempts by Trevor to use more developmentally appropriate means to have his needs met. She would be very sensitive to Trevor's nonverbal signals for communicating and look for subtle signs of distress that might indicate mounting anxiety. She would then have to make a decision to either avoid the anxiety-provoking situation or face it head on and be prepared.

At first we also had a therapist work with Trevor at home. She would simply sit beside him while he played. Interactions would be initiated by Trevor, but the therapist would watch and comment on his activities. Trevor might turn away or move to another place in the room.

The therapist would move with him and intrude on the activities again, subtly at first, then more forcefully. Once Trevor could tolerate the therapist's presence during play time, she set up games involving turn taking using puzzles, the Lego pieces, peek-a-boo, or songs involving actions.

After much persistence, Alice and the therapist realized that there were times Trevor had to take the lead and structure, even control, his mother's turn-taking play with him, to allow him to enter into the play activity. Sometimes Alice had to be a passive participant in the to and fro of social interaction. If she showed any inclination to change the pattern of play, if they did the puzzles in a different order, if they used different figurines to line up, then Trevor would get upset and go away mad. Once Alice followed her son's lead, she learned that Trevor would pay more attention to her and be more aware of her. This was an enormously important discovery for Alice and allowed her to play for longer and longer periods with her son. We could now cut back on the time for the therapist to interact with Trevor one on one. Alice gave Trevor treats like time on the computer or watching TV for playing together, for completing a puzzle with her, and for allowing her to take turns in playing with the figurines (candy is not a terrific reward since it sets up all kinds of other problems in eating and nutrition). Once she let Trevor take the lead and be more comfortable with her, it was easier to introduce modifications from within the play activity itself. An important dynamic emerged between entering Trevor's world, letting him control the agenda, and then challenging him to develop more appropriate skills. She was combining her knowledge of Trevor's inner world with some fairly standard techniques for encouraging positive behavior and learning that are used with typical children as well as children with ASD.

Trevor was easily getting twenty-five hours of therapy per week once we combined the time in day care and the sessions at home. It was nice to see that he made significant gains in the day care setting as well. Trevor started to pay more attention to his teacher. He would regularly come to her for help, would show her the newest Lego creation, his latest craft creation (which was often new pieces for his mobile). The day care introduced a picture exchange communication system (PECS), which basically allowed him to use pictures to communicate his needs. Once he developed a facility with that, his language and words appeared. He started to request food or favorite toys, then he started to label objects. His language skills made rapid progress after he learned to point to pictures or other objects of interest.

Trevor also showed more interest in the other children in day care. He would sit with them on the rotating tire in the playground. The more Trevor and the other children went to the playground together, the more his teacher had an opportunity to intrude on his happiness and get him to communicate his pleasure and enjoyment. She modeled, "Is this fun? Are you having a good time?" At first Trevor would echo these questions, but eventually he would spontaneously communicate to his teacher what fun he was having on the swings: He would smile, squeal with delight, say the word "fun," and laugh with the other children. At first this was pure verbal imitation, but soon it became part of the routine on the swings, and eventually the words and the nonverbal communications became spontaneous. By teaching some basic skills in verbal imitation, in simple skills needed to construct a theory of mind such as joint attention (where both adult and child pay attention to the same object of interest) and eye contact, the teacher could start to shape more developmentally appropriate behavior.

More and more, Trevor was able to fit in to the routine of the day care and behave just like the other children. Once Trevor learned more communication skills, both verbally and by using his pointing skills, his frustration level decreased and he became less aggressive. He did not have to resort to whacking his classmates to get them out of the way. With an outstretched arm, he could tell them to leave the room when he wanted to play with one of their toys. In addition, as his play skills improved, the periods when he would rock in the corner, flick his fingers in front of his eyes, and look autistic became farther apart. We never had to design interventions to reduce these "autistic" behaviors; they disappeared on their own as his social and communication skills improved overall.

As these positive social relationships developed at day care, the potential to use the other children in the class as "peer tutors" became possible. Trevor's teacher had to coach the other children on how to interact with Trevor, how to let him take the lead, how to avoid fights, how not to expect Trevor to share or take turns in play. But if they stuck to simple games like chasing, tag, and tickling, the other children in the class could have fun with him and they could play together. Soon Trevor sought out his classmates and wanted to play tag with them. Even more exciting was the fact that the other children were inviting Trevor to play with them. Trevor seemed to be actually enjoying the social interaction, even if it could be only at a relatively simple level. Imaginative play with his peers was beyond him at this point. That would have to await the development of further language and symbolic play skills. Alice also reported that her own parents had to learn to let Trevor take the lead, to expect little in the way of proper manners in their home, and to appreciate what little social approach he made. Her father would take Trevor to the train station, and they would look at the trains together. Trevor had always been interested in trains since he had seen Thomas the Tank Engine on TV. This gave him pleasure, and his grandfather was happy to sit on the bench at the train station and be part of this little ritual that they shared. Afterward they would go to the local coffee shop and share a hot chocolate and a doughnut.

*   *   *

Over the course of the two years of this type of intensive therapy, Trevor's improvements became more rapid, and the little victories seemed to cascade from one day to the next. Working intensively on a few pivotal skills in the social and communication domains made possible all kinds of other changes. It was like unlocking a key, only this time the key was social engagement, simple communications, imitation, and attentional flexibility and joint attention. Soon Trevor began to show an interest in the other children on the street. At first he didn't approach them, but he would respond positively if friends called on him to come out and play. Eventually he asked to see them, but only on weekends (school time was reserved for school friends). This did not happen very often, but when it did, his mother would quickly take advantage of it. Alice arranged for a little girl to come to the house on weekends and play with Trevor and watch TV.

After two years of this therapy Trevor came back for another visit. It was before his entry into kindergarten, and I had to fill in all sorts of forms for an educational assistant. I wanted to get as accurate a picture as possible of how he had done.

"I am five years old!" he announced upon entering the office.

"Are you?" I replied. "That's old. But not as old as me. Did you have a birthday party?"

"Yes, I did!"

"Who came?"

"My friends . . . from school." Now that was a reply that was worth preserving for posterity.

"Did you get any presents?"

"Yes, I did." I could see that giving longer responses was still a problem for Trevor. It was hard to get this conversation going fluidly.

"What presents did you get?"

"A mobile of stars . . . To hang over my bed."

I had to laugh. The more things change, the more they stay the same, I suppose. Even with all the work and resources that went into this amazing transformation from the toddler who ignored social interaction to the little boy who was the center of this birthday party. But it was worth it. Alice told me that as Trevor falls asleep, there are stars in his eyes. That's nice to know.

Chapter 10

Ernest
The View from the Bridge

*E*rnest is five years old. He has curly brown hair, is slightly pudgy in a cute way, and has very large brown eyes that seem to take in a lot. He loves to wear striped shirts and to visit the canal on the outskirts of town so he can spend an hour or so dropping stones off the bridge. In winter, he can become quite upset if the water ices over and the stones no longer make the sound he likes when they hit the surface. He cries, gets agitated, and sometimes will bite his hand in frustration. His parents have learned to avoid the bridge on particularly cold days, when the ice is thick. He also collects smooth pebbles at the canal's edge and takes them home, where he aligns them on his shelf in intricate patterns. Ernest enjoys playing on the computer but spends most of his time playing blackjack against it, which is remarkable given his age. His father says with some pride that if he played in a casino he would win a lot of money.

Ernest is very active, even for a five-year-old. He is so active, in fact, that he is often up at night and insists on keeping his parents awake by coming into their room, pulling off the blankets, and indicating that he wants to watch videos. As a result, they are both thoroughly exhausted—Ernest's father works frequent shifts at the local factory, and his mother has a younger child to look after. They've tried reprimanding him for this behavior, but that has had little effect, so now they have put an Etch A Sketch in his room, which he happily plays until at least 6:00 A.M., when it's time to get up for school.

Ernest is nonverbal and so has a difficult time communicating; he says nothing and never has. Some children who are unable to speak can compensate for their lack of words by signing, gesturing, or nodding and shaking their head. Ernest doesn't use any of these forms of communication except to point at objects nearby. He's quite independent and does not require his parents' help for many of his needs. He can turn on the computer and the TV by himself and can get his own food from the refrigerator. He has little desire to communicate over and above his immediate needs and wants and, for the most part, is quite content with his life. If he is denied something important, he will cry and protest and rarely, if he is extremely frustrated (like when the river freezes over), he will bite his hand. His understanding of language is also quite delayed. He does not understand, for example, why he cannot have ten Popsicles, one after another, and will have a minor temper tantrum if his intake is limited.

Ernest is enrolled in the local elementary school. He has a teacher's assistant who spends all her time just working with him under the supervision of the classroom teacher. Unfortunately they have little understanding of ASD and no experience in dealing with someone like Ernest. In spite of the fact that Ernest came to school with a diagnosis of ASD, no individual treatment or educational plan designed specifically for his needs was in place. The current plan is based on special needs children in general and says nothing about autism. This is not an uncommon occurrence; all too often schools are ill prepared to deal with the challenges of a child with ASD. As a result, Ernest is expected to follow the standard classroom routines, like sitting quietly in circle time, moving easily from activity to activity, and listening to his teacher's commands. The problem is that Ernest has a hard time sitting still (as his parents can testify and tried to tell his teachers), and he so loves the sandbox that he refuses to leave it and share it with another child. As a result, if he is not forcibly removed, he will monopolize the sandbox all day, not allowing any other child to share it and refusing to go on to other activities. If he is led away by the hand, he will hit the teacher and protest loudly. The other children look on in amazement, not understanding why he is so badly behaved.

One day Ernest bopped the teacher in the nose. Well, to be truthful, he broke her nose. It all started when he wanted to go outside. After all, it was a lovely day, one of the first days of spring, and he was keen to go on the swings. The door to the yard was locked. He started to cry and bang on the door. His teacher went over to him and tried to reason with him. But either he could not understand or he would not listen. She bent over to take his hand away from the door, and he bopped her one. The blood spurted from her nose and flowed down her expensive dress. She was crying and was very distraught, Ernest was screaming, and the entire class erupted in chaos. The teaching assistant had to go and get the principal to restore order.

Some days later a conference was held with his parents, the teacher, and the principal. Ernst was suspended and was not allowed to return until he "understood" the consequences of what he had done. He simply "had to learn that he could not always do what he wanted." He had to understand the meaning of the word "no." Ernest's parents were ashamed and humiliated. After all, what five-year-old gets suspended from elementary school? There was no one there to advocate for Ernest, to explain that he may not be able to understand the consequences of his behavior or to learn that he could not always do what he wanted. This happens all too often when assistance for special needs children is given along generic lines, without any definite attention to the needs imposed by specific disorders, such as autism. His mother had to find something else for him to do the rest of the time, which mostly meant plunking him in front of the TV or the computer so she could look after her other child. When he did return to school, the aggressive behavior seemed to increase initially, so Ernest spent more and more time at home or isolated from the other children in a room next to the principal, until thankfully the school year ended. That initial suspension ushered in a period of escalating behavioral difficulties leading to more and more suspensions. In effect, suspensions were being used as a behavior management tool.

*   *   *

There are probably few aspects of behavior in children with ASD that generate as much emotion and misunderstanding as disruptive behavior, which can include aggression toward others, yelling, self-injury, not complying with requests to do something, running away, and so on. Disruptive behavior is typical of most children with ASD, at least at some point in their development. It's true that some children tend to be passive and very compliant, but this is less common than children who show disruptive behavior in response to stress and frustration. When that frustration remains unchecked, or is not dealt with appropriately, aggression is the natural outgrowth. Aggressive behavior sets off a chain of events that leads to further problems: exclusion from community activities, increased stress in family members, and fewer opportunities for therapeutic interventions than would normally occur.

As more and more children with ASD are placed in mainstream educational settings, more and more pressure is placed on teachers to deal with aggression in the classroom. But teachers want to be teachers, not therapists. They rightly feel they should be educating children, not running a treatment center. With so many children with autism being diagnosed and going to public schools, it seems as if there are few knowledgeable consultants to help out. Teachers in the classroom are left on their own and have to rely on parents to provide guidance and direction, yet parents often feel that teachers and the schools should know how to deal with this type of problem. They are, after all, the "experts."

It's especially difficult when the aggression occurs at school but not at home or vice versa, for then there is opportunity for blaming and recrimination. It's challenging enough to deal with aggression without also feeling that one is to blame for it. In Ernest's case, his behavior was much worse at school than at home. The teachers said this was because they put more demands on him to behave "properly" and his parents should do the same at home. That way there would be more "consistency" (a favorite word for consultants who know little about children with ASD). Now Ernest's parents felt guilty as well as ashamed and humiliated.

Sometimes the opposite is true: Some children with ASD engage in more disruptive behavior at home than at school. This may be a response to severe sibling conflict, when parents cannot intervene in, or resolve, the typical sibling's resentment of the fact that the child with ASD is treated differently. (Without going into depth here, suffice it to say that when the typical sibling feels cheated by the extra attention or apparent leniency extended to the child with ASD, the solution is to make sure that the typical sibling understands why the rules are different and that he or she gets "special time" with a parent alone, doing something fun.) Much more confusing, however, are those situations where the school is so structured and regimented that the child with ASD behaves appropriately in that setting but comes home so frustrated and stressed that there is little capacity for coping with the normal stresses and strains of family life. At age seventeen, Jane was completely obsessed with Barbie dolls. When she came home from school, all she wanted to do was to dress her dolls in the same set of Barbie clothes over and over again. If she ran out of clothes, she would become so upset that she would yell and scream and throw things against the wall. The more difficulty she had at school, the more she insisted on playing with the dolls at home. If the school eased off on academic demands and gave her more free time, she was easier to handle at home. But she was never a behavior problem at school! Her disruptiveness showed only at home, in direct response to the academic demands at school. Through careful titration of the school environment and measuring of the response at home, we could develop this hypothesis and test it out systematically. When we switched Jane's program to a nonacademic one that involved more life skills, her rages at home subsided at last.

There are no easy answers to the problem of disruptive behavior, however, and sometimes extraordinary measures like medication, physical restraint, or mild reprimands are in fact required. But one tactic that should be avoided altogether is a power struggle between the child and an adult (parent or teacher). Some adults, in the face of aggression, place more limits on the child, withhold rewards, hand out minor punishments, become impatient and critical. The child senses this, and the aggressive behavior worsens in response. Thus a chain of events is set up resulting in escalating behavioral difficulties; then more limits placed on the child by the adult, which in turn leads to more aggressive behavior. Challenging behavior must never be experienced as a "challenge" that requires more control. Nobody wins a power struggle, especially when it involves a child with ASD, who has little sense that if he gave in a little, the adult might as well. The child with ASD may not understand, or be able to process quickly, that his behavior has an influence on an adult. He may just see an adult who is impatient and critical for no good reason. Aggressive behavior increases in response in large part because children with ASD cannot communicate effectively in words or do not understand intuitively why the other person will not allow them to do something. Dealing with the behavior after the fact often doesn't work; withdrawal of social attention does not have the same motivational value as it does for typical children. Children with ASD, in contrast to typical children, are never difficult because they "want attention"—such desires are generally not in their emotional vocabulary, precisely because their world revolves around a different axis, one that does not value social interaction above all else.

When aggression escalates out of control, suspension from school or a child care setting is often the end result of this struggle between child and teacher. But suspension should be used only when personal safety of the child with ASD or the other children is a real concern and only for a very limited time. At best, it allows the school an opportunity to cool off and gain some breathing space. There are few if any positive outcomes for the child. Suspension deprives the child of the opportunity to benefit from being with other children in a "normal" environment. Also, it does not work as a deterrent. Instead, it often acts to maintain the disruptive behavior because the children learn that if they misbehave they can go home and play on the computer or watch TV. For young children with autism and AS, there is a real advantage to being in an environment with other typically developing children: It provides them with the opportunity to learn appropriate social and communication skills in a natural setting.

Several studies have demonstrated the benefit of peer tutors for children with ASD. In these demonstration projects, the peers interact with the child with ASD in a supervised way under the direction of a therapist, who ensures that the activities are fun and that there are opportunities for social interaction and communication. The children with ASD can be involved in many aspects of social play appropriate to their developmental level and communication skills. Even being the center of a game such as "Ring around the Rosie" can teach the child with ASD to enjoy being close to other children rather than actively avoiding them. As a side benefit, peer tutoring gives typical children even more opportunity to be with classmates who have special needs, an experience that fosters the development of empathy and caring—an experience denied to them if the child with ASD is suspended the moment that disruptive behavior arises.

Peer interaction that benefits both the typical children and those with ASD can take place at home too; children with ASD who have younger sisters are especially lucky, since sisters are usually eager to include their older sibling in play and games. Families lucky to have lots of cousins or who live on streets with lots of children can easily take advantage of these opportunities for exposing their child with ASD to social interactions,. The more exposure a child with ASD has to social interaction, the more the opportunity to gain social and communication skills. Such activities have led to demonstrated gains in social and communication skills for some children with ASD. Other children with ASD may not yet have some of the very basic social or attending skills necessary to benefit, however, and in that case more one-on-one therapy with an adult (see Chapter 9) will be needed to prepare them for more naturalistic learning environments.

In the same way that suspension usually is not a disincentive for a child with ASD, parents learn that isolation in their rooms or extended time-outs, strategies that usually work well with typical children, do not work with children with ASD. Time-outs are good for parent relief, no doubt, and that is a worthwhile goal to be sure, but parents should not think by doing this they are teaching the child with ASD to "behave."

Some children with ASD learn to use aggression as a way of avoiding difficult situations, and to suspend them—or to send them to time-out in their room—only teaches them that they can escape these difficulties. If a child finds some academic activity difficult, whether it's listening to someone read from a book, sitting in a circle surrounded by other kids, or doing math problems, it may be easier to bop the teaching assistant than to do the assignment.

Suspending Ernest provided only temporary relief for his teacher and caused other problems for Ernest. Alternative solutions would have been more effective in dealing with the aggression as well as benefiting his overall social skills. Ernest enjoyed going to school each morning, and it had become a regular part of his routine. The other children liked playing with him and were protective toward him. They had no trouble handling Ernest; they left him alone if he was cranky and helped him if he was responsive to their ministrations. They could recognize his subtle communications more easily than his teachers, who were often too busy following the lesson plan to pay attention to his nonverbal messages of distress and frustration. Ernest's parents were also sensitive to these clues, and as a result, there was much less disruptive behavior at home.

When Ernest was finally allowed to return to school in the fall, however, he had a difficult time. His routine had been disrupted by the suspension, his opportunity to practice his social and communication skills had been reduced dramatically, and he was now treated in a guarded fashion by his teachers. Going to school was much less fun than before, and he was clearly unhappy, as it was more and more difficult for his mother to get him off to school in the morning; he would dawdle getting dressed, then resist going out the door and onto the school bus.

As behavior management strategies, suspension and "taking control" are poor options and represent desperate remedies that should be avoided if at all possible. In Ernest's case, the aggressive behavior could have been easily prevented in the first place. It was simply a matter of taking a different perspective. The key to dealing with aggression is not to focus on the aggression and violence, however difficult that might be, but to see why the behavior occurs in the first place. In Ernest's case, his difficulty was following the classroom routine. He had his own agenda and didn't understand the necessity of following anybody else's. He did not have a clue as to what the teacher was thinking or trying to do with him when she led him away from the door. Giving him a schedule that combined his favorite activities, or that allowed him to follow his own agenda with those expected of everybody else, would have been an easy solution. In children with communication difficulties, having a pictorial representation of the day's activities can be an invaluable aid in establishing such a routine. But such flexibility is all too often impractical in some classroom settings. Some institutions find it hard to have different rules for different children.

While parents quickly learn through experience and trial and error the importance of understanding the reason for disruptive or aggressive behavior, some professionals unfamiliar with ASD find this concept very difficult to accept. They are afraid of giving in, of being manipulated by a five-year-old—as if children with ASD were socially sophisticated enough to manipulate anybody, let alone someone as cagey as an adult.

The natural impulse of adults is, of course, to control a child's inappropriate behavior. But once a temper tantrum happens, there may be little chance of stopping it. Children with ASD tend to have temper tantrums that go on for a long time (perhaps because they cannot shift attention away from the object of distress), they are quite intense, and the ability to communicate or negotiate about the event (already compromised by the disability) during the tantrum is much reduced. Once a child with ASD in the middle of a tantrum reaches a point of no return, the only rule is to protect the child, protect those around him or her, and let the tantrum run its course. It is no use punishing the aggression in a vain attempt to teach the child better next time. Trying to correct past behavior is too difficult, probably because of the executive function deficits described in earlier chapters. It's much easier to teach appropriate behavior in a proactive fashion, in a positive manner, with rewards that are both tangible and immediate and coupled with social praise. That way social praise, which is intrinsically less rewarding for a child with ASD, gets paired with those tangible rewards that are highly motivating and may, by itself, become a reward later on.

It's important to enter the child's mind and, in a kind of thought experiment, experience the child with ASD's disabilities and limitations. In that way, the limited options available to that child, given the circumstances, become apparent. Once the perspective of the child is taken, all kinds of alternatives present themselves to parents and teachers, and either the recourse to disruptive behavior is avoided or else the adult helps the child find other means to satisfy that need. I remember one child who had a problem of spitting in the most inappropriate places, especially the principal's office. We could think of no way to get him to stop until we gave him some gum to chew. He preferred the gum to spitting. Another boy was particularly sensitive to loud noises and would scream whenever somebody in the neighborhood pulled out a chain saw and started sawing. The only thing that prevented the screaming was to put headphones on him and play tapes of his favorite TV shows. These are examples of providing alternatives to sensory stimulation that can be so disruptive of day-to-day functioning.

Sometimes I wistfully imagine receiving a dime for every time somebody has said to me, "His aggression is entirely unprovoked." That only tells me that people are not looking in the right places. There is always a reason for disruptive behavior. It's just that the reason may be idiosyncratic. It may be a transition that has gone unnoticed, a new smell in the classroom, a picture hanging crooked on the wall, any change in routine or the environment that causes anxiety and distress, an inability to express oneself in any other way, a social interaction that has gone awry. But unless we put ourselves in the shoes of the child, we will not be able to see this transition or this aspect of the physical and social environment as stressful. To compensate for the child's difficulties in theory of mind, we have to develop a hypertrophied theory of both our mind and the child's mind. We have to be able to infer the child's state of mind even though the child may not be able to infer ours.

Up until the suspension, Ernest was making slow but steady progress in school and was gradually becoming more comfortable with the other children. He no longer avoided them, but accepted their help in crafts and during lunch. He would look at his teaching assistant when it was time to go to the sandbox in anticipation of a fun activity. He was able to transfer his proficiency in blackjack from the computer to playing with his teaching assistant. She was most impressed with his ability to count to twenty-one! These were all considerable achievements. But his communication skills were not progressing as rapidly as his social skills. To suspend him then made little sense; it deprived him of his only treatment option, a treatment to which he was entitled. Obviously his aggression was not acceptable. But it is easy to see why it occurred and how it could have been avoided. Ernest had few communication skills available to him. He could basically protest and request—that was all.

Imagine being deprived of all forms of communication except these two. If I'm feeling particularly mischievous and cranky at a school conference, I will suggest to teachers that they pretend they can communicate only two messages; they can protest something by saying "no" or else request something by pointing. At all other times, they are to ignore the other person. Through this little thought experiment, adults soon learn to appreciate the implications of the communication disability that children with ASD have—that it involves both verbal and gestural forms of communication. It also helps them to be perhaps more sensitive to the messages that are being sent by the child. Very subtle nonverbal messages that signal mounting stress and frustration are sometimes overlooked. In Ernest's case, these included making loud sounds, flapping his arms, slamming objects on the table, and a shortening of his attention span. Paying close attention to these signals allows an adult to intervene *before* the behavior escalates into a crisis situation. Intervention in this case involved moving on to another activity that Ernest found more enjoyable and then back to the more demanding task. This turned out to be a much more effective way of dealing with his behavior and led to more opportunities for learning in the classroom.

Aggression is always a communication. It's a signal of distress that cannot be communicated except through aggressive behavior, either because the child is nonverbal or because he does not understand the meaning of a social interaction. The key to treatment is either to provide the child with an alternative form of communication or else to intuit what the child is communicating and respond appropriately. When adults understand the function a disruptive behavior serves, why it occurs in the first place, and are able to change the environment so that it is less stressful, the child learns the value of communicating, and this awareness fosters the development of his own communication skills.

Aggression is often reduced when children with autism learn to use augmentative forms of communication such as pictures, form boards, or signs. When Ernest went back to school in the fall, he had a new consultant who was quite knowledgeable about ASD. She suggested that the teachers use a picture exchange system as an augmentative form of communication. She also suggested that a visual schedule of the day's activities be placed somewhere in the classroom so that the teacher could show Ernest it was time to move on to another activity. She also recommended that the first activity of the day be time on the computer in class. That would ensure that Ernest looked forward to coming into class and was in a good mood at the start of the day. Difficult activities were interspersed with more fun activities, even if this meant that Ernest was on a different schedule than the other children in the classroom. If needed, when those nonverbal signals of frustration began to escalate, Ernest could have some quiet time, outside the classroom, for short periods of time, but then a quick return to classroom activities would ensure that he would not learn how to avoid schoolwork. No punishments were administered, and the criteria for suspensions were clearly spelled out. But once these initiatives were in place, there was never any need for suspension.

I saw Ernest some time later, and it was clear that he had taken to the picture symbols readily. When he wanted to go outside, he simply retrieved the picture for outside and showed it to his parents or teacher. If going outside was impossible, Ernest was shown the appropriate sign, a simple "Stop" sign that he would have seen all the time with his parents driving to the bridge. He seemed to understand the meaning of "no" perfectly well if it was presented to him in a visual format rather than in a verbal way. The teachers learned that he was not being stubborn when he did not respond to verbal requests but only that he was having trouble processing verbal instructions. The frequency of disruptive and more serious aggressive behavior decreased dramatically, and as a result, Ernest made much more rapid progress in that one year with a specific program for him than he did the years before, when suspension was a common occurrence. He started using the picture system at home as well; he started asking his parents for help more often; and he engaged in more social play with his younger sister, playing tag and hide and seek.

Sometimes it is much more difficult to discern the reasons for disruptive behavior. Thought experiments that imagine the world from the perspective of the child with ASD are not always initially successful and may require diligent effort on everybody's part. Even with the best of intentions, the mind of the child or adolescent with ASD can remain opaque, with troubling consequences, but to respond to disruptive behavior with suspension and "zero tolerance" is to completely misunderstand the meaning of having special needs, the responsibility we all share to preserve diversity. It is to exclude the child from a therapeutic setting, to expel the most vulnerable members of a community. It is to see "evil" where none exists, to be punitive where kindness and grace are required instead. To suspend diminishes both the child and the institution, whether it's a preschool, a high school, a recreation center, or a camp. Suspension makes vengeance a legitimate strategy of dealing with those who, because of their biological destiny, cannot follow the rules of the institutions we employ to socialize our children. Aggression is a serious problem, that is true, but to meet violence with suspension is simply to be aggressive in return. It turns having a disability into a moral issue, the educational equivalent of sin, of being "cast out." Maybe Ernest was right to be disruptive in that classroom setting. It served to warn us that institutions sometimes lack a theory of mind as well, and that these same institutions have to build bridges to families and children with ASD, not expect them to cross the river unaided.

Chapter 11

Frankie
Learning and Forgetting at School

*F*rankie was very smart. His IQ was 125, he started reading at age three, and he knew the capitals of all the countries in Europe by the time he was five. In day care he was known as the "little professor." His parents, Mike and Daphne, who were both academics, expected great things of him in school, and at first they were not disappointed. His early school years were largely trouble free since he could rely on his reading skills to get by. He could recite the alphabet before anyone else in class; he could count to fifty before anyone else could get to ten. He quickly learned all the flags of the world. He was the marvel of the local school, and all the teachers talked about how bright he was, especially since they knew he had a diagnosis of AS. But now Frankie was in grade three, and he was languishing near the bottom of the class. It was not that he did not have the ability; everybody recognized his talents. The problem was that Frankie was obsessed with flags of the world, and this obsession consumed all his interest and his attention. He knew the colors of every country's flag and its design and would pore over flag books for hours. He had a remarkable memory for these types of visual designs. But in class he was learning nothing of the standard curriculum.

What had been cute at age four was now annoying. His teachers complained that one day he would learn something and the next he would forget it. He rarely paid attention, often wandered around the room and stared out the window, looking at the flag in the schoolyard. Instead of answering questions in class, he asked questions about the colors of various flags seen around town.

"What are the colors of the flag at city hall? What about the flag at the car dealership?" he would ask with a grin.

Though his teachers knew perfectly well that Frankie knew the answers to these questions, they would patiently answer them. This did not, however, reduce the frequency of the questioning. By the end of the day, Frankie could become quite aggressive if his questions were not answered immediately. Sometimes he would hit the other children, throw books on the floor, have screaming fits. His teachers reluctantly suggested to his parents that they consider home schooling. The school board would be happy to provide him with a tutor.

Frankie's situation was becoming desperate. His parents came to see me, hoping I could find a way to improve his behavior and his learning at school. To teach him at home would mean depriving him of the opportunity to interact with other children and so perhaps improve his social interactions. Frankie had enjoyed his first school years and had made some friends who came to the house to play and invited him to their birthday parties in return. The more time Frankie spent with other children, the less he seemed to pursue his eccentric interests at home. Now he wanted to play with other children, not just on his own. His parents thought this positive change was a product of their determination that he go to the local school rather than to a special school for children with autism. But now he was clearly unhappy in school; he was bored and uninterested in the regular school subjects and was interested only in flags. He was making little progress in reading and arithmetic. He showed no inclination toward social studies or science. His teachers said his autistic symptoms and his obsession with flags were preventing him from learning the curriculum and were interfering with the education of the other students. Those children no longer wanted to come over to his house to play. Because he was so bright, the teachers assumed that he could learn the regular curriculum in the usual way.

I have known Frankie since early childhood. He was always interested in things that blow in the wind. I remember his mother telling me that when she hung laundry out to dry on blustery mid-summer mornings, Frankie would run back and forth laughing gleefully as the wind made the sheets billow from side to side. He loved to go to the park and fly kites with his father—great big blue kites with long tails that swished back and forth, dove into the wind, and then caught an updraft and sailed straight up into the sky. All this was charming and amusing, and it gave him and his parents much joy and pride. But now his interest in things that blow in the wind was causing considerable distress and making it difficult for Frankie to learn anything at school. He was in danger of being marginalized and excluded from his school community.

*   *   *

One of the challenges that teachers face in dealing with children with autism and AS is that it's difficult to get their attention or to motivate them to do any schoolwork. They are generally not interested in following the standard curriculum—in learning math facts, writing an essay, or playing with other children in the schoolyard. A teacher standing at the head of the class will not catch the attention of a child like Frankie. He will not necessarily look at the teacher, process what the teacher is saying, or follow directions. Frankie may be daydreaming, replaying in his mind certain cartoons or movies he saw years ago, remembering the video game he played last night, or mentally running though the collection of flags he has at home. His body is there, but his mind is somewhere else. What takes place in the social context of the classroom does not have meaning in a compelling way for the child with ASD.

The other difficulty is that the learning style of a child with ASD is different from that of more typical children. Frankie has a prodigious memory for facts and for visual details. It may take him a while to learn something, but when he does, he learns it very well. The problem is that he cannot generalize from the facts to more abstract or conceptual rules; he has difficulty categorizing his experiences and his learning. So, for example, Frankie can learn how to solve a mathematical word problem involving apples and oranges but not if the same concept is presented as shoes and socks. He can learn about the meaning of a word such as "history" by reference to early settlers to this country but not in reference to early settlers in South America. He can learn why it's wrong to hit a child because he has taken something that belongs to him but cannot apply it when the other child will not share a toy. He can learn specific rules but cannot always apply those rules to new situations.

At home, Frankie's parents had learned that everything has to be broken down into component parts and each part taught in detail. The parts then have to be assembled one by one into a new concept. His parents had to teach him how to brush his teeth by taking pictures of each step involved in the process: picking up the toothbrush, putting toothpaste on the brush, brushing his teeth, and spitting into the sink. Once each step was taught individually, he had to learn to do them in sequence. But at the end of it all, he was better and more consistent at brushing his teeth than his brothers and sisters!

The other problem is that catching Frankie's interest in academic activities is even more difficult than for typical children. What motivates and interests Frankie are the capitals of Europe, flags of the world, stamps (but only those with flags on them), and old maps; he is simply not interested in the typical things that an eight-year-old is interested in, such as sports, the latest Japanese animation, robots, and transformers. So when other children come over to his house to play, Frankie wants to show them his collection of flags, which is interesting to them for about fifteen minutes. The other children then want to play with Frankie's neglected toys—the cars and the electric train set. Frankie stays in his room, poring over his books and ignoring his friends. His parents sigh in frustration and wonder what to do. Soon the friends stop coming over.

But sometimes children with ASD are in schools that are able to capitalize on their extraordinary capacity for visual learning. When this happens, gifted and creative teachers can make learning and participation in school both therapeutic and an opportunity for growth. The teacher is able to see the autistic disability as a gift, as a talent to be exploited, not as a symptom to be eliminated. This insight comes from a profound respect for the mind of the child with ASD and an intuitive capacity for understanding and imagining the mind of other people. Not all unusual interests can be transformed in such a way, but when it does happen, the potential for learning is remarkable. It is also true that these schools and teachers are hard to find, but they do exist. The best way to find schools that are flexible in their approach to a child with ASD is to see if the school has had previous experience with ASD, if it has used the consultants and experts it has available to it, and if the school has enjoyed working with children with ASD. Schools that see these children as a burden, as extra work, are to be avoided if possible. Many boards have special teams that will consult with specific schools about a child with ASD in that classroom and help design an educational program that takes that child's learning style into account. A principal and teacher that listen to these local experts and implement the recommendations in the classroom are the best schools for children with ASD. Just because a child has an Individualized Education Plan (IEP) does not mean that the school has the expertise or willingness to take these learning styles into account. A child can have the best individualized program in his educational folder, but if the plan is not implemented with the assistance of experts it is unlikely that the plan will be used effectively. Willingness to learn and to accept new challenges are the most important predictors of success. These schools see parents as an important part of the education team, not as potential critics to be held at a distance. They use reports sent home to tell good stories about the child's day at school, not all the bad things that happened. I remember one school where the teacher wrote things like "Teresa should learn not to pass gas in class." This is an example of a school unwilling to work with parents in a constructive fashion. If parents have a choice about what school their child may attend, it is worthwhile to compare and contrast several schools and choose the one with the most experience with children with ASD or the one most willing to be flexible and accommodating and one that treats parents as part of the team.

* * *

We had a school conference for Frankie that turned out quite well, in fact. The principal and teacher were genuinely interested in learning how to help Frankie and were willing to listen to their special education consultants—a psychologist, a special education teacher, and a speech pathologist—all of whom had experience with children with ASD and were aware of the latest research on learning styles in this population. The special education teacher, who attended Frankie's conference, had many helpful things to say. She understood that the key was not to make Frankie follow the standard curriculum, not to focus on what he could not do, but rather to capitalize on his particular strengths and talents—his memory for details, his ability to see patterns and to decode complex visual figures (like letters and numbers) into simpler parts. Focusing on the ways in which these children can learn is much more effective than focusing on what they cannot do.

The consultant suggested that Frankie's teacher use his interest in flags as a vehicle for learning about math; if you have two flags and you multiply by another five, how many flags will you have? Frankie could picture this scenario in his mind without difficulty, and it turned out to be much easier to teach Frankie math this way, rather than using the traditional examples in the books. She also suggested that Frankie would be able to read more fluently by giving him material about flags of the world: flags from different times in history, flags used for different purposes. Soon Frankie's interests expanded to heraldry as a direct result of the readings she supplied, which led to all sorts of possibilities and was enormous fun for him and his classmates. Not long afterward, Frankie was drawing heraldry designs for his friends, and they were plastering them all over the school. Each class became a different castle with its own coat of arms. Eventually, this changed into an interest in knights of old, and Frankie and his friends started playing at his house for hours as knights of the round table, pretending to slay dragons and rescuing fair maidens.

I also remember Ben, who was fascinated with sports statistics. He would wake up at 6:00 A.M. every morning, and the first thing he would do is go downstairs and turn on the sports channel to find out the latest scores. He could recite the score of every game, including from some sports that nobody seemed to care about (like Australian-rules football and fourth division English soccer). During the winter of his second grade at school, his teacher asked him to tell everybody in class the score of the latest Toronto Maple Leafs hockey game. Now, in Canada, this made him an instant celebrity. Soon he was publishing a small newspaper on the computer at school, writing stories about all his favorite hockey players, calculating various statistics (including "goals against" average), and presenting this information to his classmates. The other boys in the class found this fascinating and started to spend more time with him. Eventually he made some friends who came over to the house, and they started a Maple Leafs fan club in their neighborhood. All this was facilitated by Ben's teacher, who allowed him to pursue his interests in class instead of the standard curriculum as set out in the lesson plans. He learned the same material but did it in his own way, using his own interests and obsessions. Such gifted teachers are uncommon, but with the rules and regulations concerning special education and the necessity of individualized educational programs, there is more and more opportunity for these kinds of creative avenues as a teacher. In these types of learning environments, Frankie and other children with ASD can become motivated, will pay attention in class, and will be interested in going to school. By modifying the learning curriculum to take account of a child's eccentric interests and preoccupations, it is possible to educate children with ASD more effectively.

Eccentric interests and preoccupations represent activities with a high motivational value, ways of getting the child's attention and of promoting more social interaction with adults and with other children. By starting with the child's interests and building on them, it is also possible to promote more appropriate social and communication skills. For example, many children with autism love to watch a top spin. The enjoyment elicited by this activity can become a vehicle for social interaction: An adult spins the top; several children can participate in the activity; they can take turns spinning the top; the teacher or parent can talk about the colors and can demonstrate pleasure as the top spins; the teacher or parent can encourage the child to ask for help in spinning and use words like "fast" and "slow" to describe the speed of spin, and so on. The child is motivated to participate, happy and excited. It is an opportunity to enter the child's world at his or her own level and to bring the child up a developmental notch. This is incidental learning in a natural environment, and it is a very effective form of teaching for some children with ASD.

There was a time when Heather (the little girl with the bathing suit from Chapter 2) was having a very hard time going to school. She put up a lot of resistance from the moment she woke up all the way to the schoolyard. She would dawdle getting dressed, stop and look at every broken twig along the way, and then stand still before the school entrance, refusing to go in. Once in the class, she would hide under the desk and make a racket to force the teacher to send her to the principal's office, where she would be put in a "quiet" room for a while, then forced back into the classroom or, if she was unruly, sent home. This was becoming a real problem, with Heather being sent home more and more often, which made it very difficult for her mother, the sole breadwinner, to be available at work. At a school meeting, her mother suggested that the teacher let Heather design Easter cards first thing in the school day, as she loved greeting cards of every type. This was a highly motivating activity for Heather at home, where she spent hours drawing different kinds of cards, depending on the time of year. Perhaps, if she were given an opportunity to draw cards, she would find it easier to go to school in the morning and would arrive in a better mood and be more attentive to learning.

So during the week, as soon as Heather woke up, her mother would start telling her that at school she would be able to draw Easter cards first thing before starting class. Heather looked at her mother quizzically, not believing her good luck. Each day that week, Heather worked in her private space, drawing all kinds of Easter cards, making one for each child in the class and one for her teacher and principal.

This she did attentively and with great enthusiasm. Now her mother had no trouble getting Heather to go to school. She woke up and got ready for school without incident. Broken twigs still attracted her attention, but there was no resistance at the entrance to the school, no hanging on to the doors as she was being pulled into class. Each day, she worked industriously on her cards, and when they were all done she handed them out to all the children in the class. She was beaming with pride, and of course the other children were thrilled to get these early Easter cards—it was, after all, just March. The teacher was a little apprehensive as to what Heather could work on next, but it turned out that after Easter there is Mother's Day, Father's Day, and so on. In fact the greeting card industry has arranged it so that there are holidays needing cards all year long! What luck! All this activity put Heather in a better mood, and she was quite happy in class—no more hiding under the desk, making funny noises, being abrasive and difficult with the teacher or her teacher's aide. In fact, she was in such a good mood that she was able to make real progress in reading and basic arithmetic, a major accomplishment that year.

* * *

Harry walked into the office one day rather proudly, bearing the picture of a fish on his T-shirt. I asked him if he liked fish. "Oh, yes," he said, "very much." Did he own fish at home? "Oh, yes, we have a fifty-gallon tank with lots of fish," he said. What was his favorite fish? "A puffer fish," he said. What kind was it? I asked. "Puffer fish live in the tropical and subtropical parts of the Atlantic, Indian, and Pacific Oceans. There are about one hundred twenty species of puffer fish," he replied, not quite answering my question but leaving me impressed with his knowledge of fish.

Harry was fifteen years old. He had dark hair down to his shoulders that often covered his eyes. He would look at me with his head down, not quite, but almost, avoiding eye contact. He always wore T-shirts with pictures of tropical fish stenciled on them. He loved animals, especially scaly ones, and he knew an extraordinary amount about the history and breeding of various fish and reptiles. He had at least fifty stuffed reptiles, dinosaurs, and fish covering his bed. They all had to be arranged in perfect order before he went to sleep. While this was very cute, it was perhaps a little inappropriate for a teenager. In fact, his classmates teased him quite mercilessly for his immaturity.

Harry was originally referred to me with a diagnosis of "nonverbal learning disability." This label refers to children with good reading and language skills but poor academic achievement in math, poor fine and gross motor coordination, and poor drawing skills. Nonverbal learning disabilities contrast with the classic dyslexia type of reading disability, where the children show poor academic achievement in reading, phonics, and (often but not always) mathematics in spite of good overall intelligence and an adequate opportunity for learning. The problem was that as time went on, Harry was falling farther and farther behind his classmates in the more difficult subjects in high school. The main problem now was one of organization; he could not work independently, wandered around the classroom, could not start his homework, felt easily overwhelmed by projects. He was also more and more isolated from his peers and was unhappy about the fact that they were all going out with girls and he was left alone at home with his parents and the fish tank!

Harry, in fact, behaved in ways consistent with AS; the learning disability was just part of the problem. His early history noted that he was always isolated, tended to play by himself and avoid inviting his parents into his play, had poor conversation skills, was never very chatty, and was fascinated with animals. He used to line up his stuffed toys from his bedroom into the living room and down the stairs into the basement. He was, however, able to read at three years of age. His mother remembers him reading from his father's textbooks (he was an accountant) by the time he was five. He loved to read and even to this day loves chapter books, though they are often of an immature variety designed to appeal to younger readers. He did well in school until grade four, then started to have problems with math. A psychological assessment revealed the classic profile of a nonverbal learning disability, and he started to receive some extra help. But by high school he was finding it more and more difficult to keep up not only in math but in all his subjects. The difficulty was especially evident in subjects that required lots of homework and independent study projects.

It is not uncommon for children with AS to get a diagnosis of nonverbal learning disability. The two overlap but are not identical. Nonverbal learning disability is a diagnosis based on performance on academic tests and overall intelligence; it does not involve problems with social skills or communication or obsessive interests. Many children with AS have this cognitive profile, but not all do. In addition, there are many children with nonverbal learning disability who do not have AS. Nevertheless the confusion continues in the literature.

Once we cleared up the diagnosis, Harry's parents wanted some help on instructional strategies to improve his school performance. To do this, it was important to explain to them the kinds of difficulties that children with ASD demonstrate in cognitive testing. This subject has been researched thoroughly, and the results are fairly consistent. In fact, some researchers see autism as primarily an information-processing disorder, a convincing explanation as long as that includes the processing of social information as well.

The most common finding in ASD is a discrepancy between verbal and nonverbal cognitive skills; that is, children with autism are said to have good nonverbal skills and poor verbal skills. This is reflected in their scores on IQ tests, where the verbal scores are often well below their nonverbal scores, based on tests of matching, copying, pattern recognition, rote memory, and so on. As mentioned earlier, children with AS may have the opposite pattern: good verbal and relatively poor nonverbal skills. This may seem paradoxical given that both are forms of ASD. In fact, perhaps a better explanation of cognitive difficulties in ASD than the verbal–nonverbal discrepancy is provided by differentiating rote skills from the more complex skills of integration and using contextual cues. Children with ASD (both those with autism and those with AS) tend to have relatively good rote skills, whether in the verbal or nonverbal domains. That is why somebody like Harry was able to read at such an early age: He had excellent rote skills in both visual–spatial processing (so he could recognize groups of letters and organize them into sounds and syllables) and basic rote verbal skills (so he could sound the letters out). It was true that he couldn't understand much of what he read, but his ability to sound out the letters and syllables was excellent. As a result, Harry and other children with ASD often have good word recognition skills but poor comprehension of a paragraph or a sentence. As long as the task is simple and relies on rote skills, the child is able to learn easily. But as the children develop, performance on more complex tasks (whether verbal or nonverbal) falls off more rapidly in children with ASD than in typically developing children. This leads to an inefficiency in learning, poor use of contextual clues to understand a problem, and a failure to use organizing strategies to process new information. In other words, children with ASD find it difficult to learn by rote in one situation and apply it to another. This is probably the result of the deficits in executive function or in switching attention among children with ASD referred to earlier.

Instructional strategies, therefore, need to take advantage of these relative strengths in rote learning and apply them to situations where learning requires more complex organizing principles. Since visual presentation of learning materials is often simpler than verbal presentation, picture symbols, photographs, drawings, and other graphics are effective ways to teach children with ASD. These visual clues help organize the child. They allow the teacher to break a complex task down into component parts, deal with each part in isolation, then combine them in a rote way to accomplish the more complex demands of learning. We taped a "process" sheet to Harry's desk to remind and cue him on how to work independently: If it was a homework assignment, step 1 was to underline each component of the assignment, step 2 to make notes for each part, step 3 to type them together in one paragraph, and step 4 to edit the paragraph to improve the flow. He needed reminders of this process each time he did his homework and initially required a tutor to take him step by step through the routine. Eventually, the tutor could fade out at the end of the process and not prompt him. But Harry always needed help to get started, to sit down, look at the sheet, and start to beak down the homework assignment into its parts. The key difference between Harry and his classmates was that in addition to needing to be taught the content of his classes, he needed to be taught how to organize his work, how to solve a problem. Every class assignment, whether it was reading, writing, mathematics, history, or science, had to be reformulated so that the learning could be initiated by rote and could bypass his weaker organizing strategies.

An easier way to accomplish this is often through computer-assisted instruction. Children with ASD love to use computers, and will happily stay on them for hours. In fact, it is often so difficult to get them off the computer that it almost seems like an addiction. Fortunately, there are now many programs on the computer that can teach young children with ASD to read and do simple math operations. Several studies have shown that children with ASD learn faster by computer than through verbal instruction, perhaps because the computer not only holds their attention longer but also uses the principle of presentation by visual means, which is less complex and requires less contextual cuing to be understood. Computer-assisted instruction made a huge difference to Zachary (Chapter 4) in his early school years. He learned to read and do addition, subtraction, and basic multiplication all by computer, using only the commercially available programs. All these programs work by breaking down the complex task of reading or other subject matter into its component parts. In the case of reading, the child practices over and over again the symbol-to-sound correspondence and practices putting together the sounds into words and eventually into sentences.

* * *

Understanding the way children with ASD think is a large part of the "art" of teaching them in schools. Indeed, this understanding is a prerequisite to learning since it provides a framework for understanding the goals of an education and where to begin, and suggests the ways to achieve those goals. In supportive environments, both Frankie and Heather were capable of learning a great deal. Yet the process of learning for them is not the same as it is for typical children, and it is precisely this recognition (and the ensuing accommodation on the part of parents and teachers) that allowed such positive skills to develop. What Frankie's teacher and Heather's mother were able to appreciate was the advantage of using eccentric interests as a vehicle for learning the standard curriculum, the need to break down the complex into the simple, to use rote learning skills to learn these more simple concepts, and to use visual presentations of educational concepts (especially computers) to enhance understanding. This approach, it is important to understand, is primarily an accommodation to the disorder, not a treatment of it, based on understanding the disorder in all its myriad manifestations. Such strategies will not erase the deficits that come with ASD, but they will help prevent those deficits from making it impossible for the child to learn. When teachers and parents capitalize on a child's strengths and work around the child's deficits, provide a positive and supportive environment for learning, and hold appropriate expectations for the child given the learning characteristics of a child with ASD, the child can enjoy going to school just as much as typical children. An added benefit of that enjoyment is that social and communication skills improve as well.

I sometimes walk to the apple orchard that overlooks the station where Trevor and his grandfather watch the trains come and go (see Chapter 9). I sit very still on the old bench at the top of the hill. The wind blows through the trees and causes the long grass to change color as the breeze travels up the hillside. I remember Frankie and his kites.

He gets such enjoyment from a wind like this. It gives him an opportunity to fly that kite way up in the sky, plunging and sailing with what looks like wild abandon. It's gratifying to see him now, so much happier at school. The school appreciates his talents, ignores his eccentricities that are irksome, and in general accommodates but, at the same time, challenges him. Heather, too, finally has found a school environment that appreciates her talents, and she is now enjoying that walk to school in the morning. These developments contrast starkly with those dark days when going to school was a little hell both for them and for their parents, when they were at odds with the institution of school, when there was no understanding of ASD, when there was no accommodation to their talents and eccentricities.

*   *   *

There is a remarkable short story by Jorge Luis Borges, the Argentinean writer, that perfectly illustrates what happens when there is no accommodation to a child's difficulties. The story is called "Funes, the Memorious," about a young man with a prodigious memory who can forget nothing. He remembers every detail of his life in the particulars and is completely absorbed in his contemplation of the visible world. He is acutely aware of the uniqueness of everything he sees and so cannot categorize or generalize; a dog seen at one time of the day is not the same dog seen a minute later. And, in fact, he is right, as the pre-Socratics would have said. His learning style lacks organizational strategies, lacks the ability to use contextual cues to categorize and apply one concept to several situations. Funes's memory challenges our conventional notion of what is unique and what is different, what is the same and what is a repetition. But it comes at a cost, obviously, and that is the difficulty in learning and thinking: "To think is to forget a difference, to generalize, to abstract," writes Borges. And because Funes could not forget, he could not generalize. The narrator of the story is profoundly affected by his night of conversation with Funes: "It occurred to me that each one of my words (each one of my gestures) would live on in his implacable memory; I was benumbed by the fear of multiplying superfluous gestures." Funes is paralyzed by the multiplicity of superfluous gestures that infect his memory, and his cognitive system quickly becomes overloaded as he remembers everything and forgets nothing, just like the child with ASD.

This short story captures very nicely the inner world of children with ASD, their prodigious memory, their fascination with the visible, their love of facts and details, but also their difficulty with inferring something from what is *not* seen and the difficulty in generalization, abstraction, and conceptual thought. It is important to understand this learning style, this way of seeing the world so as to teach children with ASD at school. Both Frankie's teacher and Janice, Heather's mother, had an intuitive understanding of this and were able to capitalize on their knowledge to enter the world of the child they were working with and challenge that child to reach up to another developmental level. The key was not to expect Frankie and Heather to follow the standard curriculum or the usual parenting guidelines, but for adults to first adapt to the child's way of thinking and *then* move the child along his or her own developmental pathway.

What must it be like to remember all the flags of the world, all the flags around town? Frankie solemnly tells me that each flag is different. I suppose that is true, but my memory is not good enough to visualize these differences in any detail. I hear Frankie's voice asking me, in a gently mocking tone, if I am the same person who sat here last week in this apple orchard or a different one. As I get up to walk home, I resolve not to make any superfluous gestures. It is very difficult, but once I master it, even for a moment, the atmosphere becomes very still. I imagine that Frankie and Heather already know such stillness when they look at and discern the patterns that are invisible to us. They already know the rule about superfluous gestures. No school had to teach them that.

Chapter 12

Sophie
Acceptance without Resignation

*D*own the main street of a small village, a little girl and her mother go to the library. They make this brief excursion every day because the child so loves to look at books. It's a fine autumn morning, and the sun shines brightly as the two walk down a street shaded by oak and maple trees. Soon it will be Halloween, and already the houses are decorated with pumpkins and witches on broomsticks. The maple trees are in full color—red, yellow, and orange leaves filter the sunlight. An elderly gentleman rakes the fallen leaves on his lawn into tidy piles, but the slight breeze is a constant challenge, teasing his efforts and delaying the opportunity to go back into the house and make another pot of coffee. As the couple passes by, the man says, "Good morning," tips his hat, and smiles at the child. The mother politely, if somewhat awkwardly, returns his greeting, but the child looks away and doesn't acknowledge him.

The mother has a few volumes to be returned tucked under her arm. She wears a light sweater to guard against the wind and a lovely print dress. She has very fair skin and dark hair. The mother looks anxiously down at her child, who walks as if determined not to waste any time. The little girl must be about five; she has an olive complexion, wears glasses, and has soft curly brown hair. She is dressed all in red, her favorite color. In one hand she holds several bird feathers and in the other an enormous tree branch that she drags along the ground. People passing by have to step out of the way to avoid being hit by one of the branches. The mother tries not to look embarrassed, but this is a small town, and everybody knows that little Sophie, who was adopted from a Romanian orphanage, is a bit "unusual." She takes tree branches with her everywhere, and only with the greatest reluctance will she put them down outside the library or her house. She never says hello or returns a greeting. At the library, she refuses the librarian's help, rushes to the same bookshelf, and takes down the same book day after day—the story of a little girl who always likes to wear red clothes. If, for some reason, the book is not available, Sophie becomes upset and starts to run around the library until the librarian can find another book full of pictures of red things. Her mother often has to chase after her daughter to avoid disrupting the other patrons. When Sophie leaves the library with her mother, she picks up the tree branch outside the building and walks home, looking for other feathers or sticks. If she sees something that catches her fancy, she will drop whatever she is carrying and pick that up instead. She always has something in her hands. Her mother is relieved to be going home to make lunch. She looks forward to dropping Sophie off at the child development center in town that afternoon and having a bit of a rest.

* * *

Greg and Marianne led a comfortable and prosperous life. She was a civil servant and he worked as a land registrar. They were sweethearts in high school and stayed together through college and various job positions, eventually settling down in a small town within commuting distance of a large urban center. Long ago they decided not to have children. They liked the freedom and added income that not having children allowed them. Greg and Marianne have lived in this small town for more than ten years. They have made lots of friends, enjoyed giving parties at their house and chatting with the neighbors. They took trips to Europe every two years and often went into the city to go shopping.

In 1990, as the Communist regime was crumbling, reports came out of Romania describing the deplorable conditions in the orphanages. Greg and Marianne happened to watch a show on TV with pictures of babies in cribs, tiny infants who were dirty, crying, with their heads shaven, lying listless in filthy cots. Marianne decided they should try to adopt one of these babies. The reasons behind this decision were not clear to her or to Greg. It is not that any maternal light went on, they

were not particularly religious, they were not committed to changing
the world or to saving the earth's children out of some sense of duty. Instead, the sight of dying children made them think of their own death:
"I didn't want to think I could have done something but didn't. I did not
want to have any regrets when I died. Adoption was a way of doing
something useful. Who wants another one of *us* anyway?" Marianne explained to me one day. The only stipulation they made in their own
minds was not to adopt a baby, because it was difficult to test for AIDS,
or a child with a handicap, as that would have been overwhelming.

Eventually they were approved for an adoption by the Canadian
authorities but had no definite plans to go to Romania. One day, they
heard almost by chance on the radio that the Romanian government
was intending to limit foreign adoptions. If they did not make a move
now, they might not be able to adopt at all. Within forty-eight hours,
Marianne was on a flight to Bucharest. She had to be there by Sunday,
choose a child within a few days, complete all the paperwork, and be
home the following week.

Bucharest was filled with North Americans looking to adopt children as the government was teetering on the brink of collapse. At the
airport, each prospective parent was assigned an interpreter. Finding ac-
commodations was a problem as there was no room at any of the hotels
and Marianne did not have a chance to make a reservation from Canada. Many of the interpreters rented their own apartment to the North
Americans, demanding rates higher than hotels would have charged.
The interpreter, a woman of slight build and old-fashioned clothes, was
kind enough to take Marianne to her own apartment in the city and not
expect these exorbitant prices. Marianne was shocked to see how pov-
erty-stricken the interpreter was; the apartment was filthy, the couches
were overstuffed and torn, light bulbs without shades hung loosely
from the ceiling, there were streaks of grime on the walls, the wallpaper
was bulging from wet spots in the structure behind it. Marianne was left
alone while the interpreter went to find a child to be adopted. Only the
mice scratching in the kitchen kept her company, unconcerned by any
human intruder.

After three days the interpreter came back and told Marianne about
a "beautiful baby" she had found. She was "gorgeous, very smart and
very intelligent. Would Mrs. like to see her?"

"Yes, of course. What do you know about her?" The interpreter replied that the three-year-old child, whose name was Sophie, had lived

for the last two years in Bucharest #1, a large orphanage in the center of town. Marianne had seen the building on the cab ride from the airport. It was a huge, imposing building, with large shutters and no greenery. It had struck Marianne that it could pass for the headquarters of the secret police. Instead it was "home" to hundreds of babies and children, most with little hope of adoption. Marianne remembered the pictures from TV. Each floor contained many cribs all lined up in rows. The children lay in cots, were rarely taken out into the sunshine or out to play. Children from the poorest families and those of gypsy origin were usually placed at the back of the room, where they received even less attention than those at the front, nearest the nursing station. Marianne learned from the interpreter that the child's mother was a gypsy who gave up the baby soon after birth.

The next day, the interpreter brought Sophie, wrapped in a blanket, to the apartment. Marianne was shocked when she saw her. The child was shaking and covered in sores. Her head had been shaved in an attempt to prevent lice, and she was still in a diaper. She could not lift her head up and was covered in diarrhea that had leaked around the diaper. She weighed about fifteen pounds and looked emaciated. The interpreter asked if Marianne wanted to feed her. She handed Marianne a giant pop bottle with an agricultural nipple on it as Sophie could not yet chew solids. The bottle contained milk of indeterminate age and color. Sophie had a hard time sucking, and Marianne noticed that she kept her eyes turned to one side. Marianne tried to talk to her, but still Sophie would not look at her.

Marianne had brought some toys for the child to play with. While at the airport waiting for her assigned interpreter, she had talked to other parents, who had given her advice about toys that could be used to assess a child's level of intelligence. Sophie was placed on the carpet, propped up by pillows, and Marianne arranged the toys close by. But Sophie did not play with them. She felt them, turned them around in her hand, and brought them up close to her eyes. She was alert but very distant. Marianne tried to relate to her, to talk to her. But Sophie, with sores all over and shaking from head to toe, was in her own world. Other adoptive parents had told Marianne that the "smart ones" create another world for themselves as a protection. It would take Sophie a long time to come out of her world, if she ever came out at all, Marianne thought. She looked down at Sophie and said to herself, "You were exactly what we decided not to adopt."

It was at that moment that Greg called, excited. "Well?" he asked.

"We can't take her. You have never seen a child like this. She is not a child; she has no soul."

"What do you mean?" Greg asked incredulously. He could not understand. Marianne told him how horrible Sophie looked, how she did not talk, could not walk, and was in her own world. If they adopted her, they would have to forget all their plans about the future; in fact there would be no future. They would just be in a prison, caring for this profoundly damaged child. They would have nothing left over for themselves.

Greg listened patiently, thought for a moment, and then asked, "Why don't you take her?" Marianne protested again, describing what Sophie looked like, the sores, the shaking, the shaved head. "We can't. It's too impossible." But the more Marianne protested, the more she realized that she had to take her. "Where would she go back to? Shit, she would die back in that orphanage," she said over the phone. Then Marianne started to cry, heaving sobs, weeping for this poor child, staring at some pathetic toy on the carpet of this filthy apartment in the middle of a city on the verge of disintegration, watched over by an interpreter, who smiled benightedly at this poor strange woman, heaving with grief by the phone.

Greg whispered, ten thousand miles away, but as close as if he were beside her, "Just take her. Just take her. Promise me, will you?"

* * *

The paperwork to get Sophie out of Romania was prodigious. Marianne hired a good lawyer, and they went to court to get the papers signed. Marianne was interviewed as to whether she would make a good mother. Sophie was also examined by the doctors. She had not been out of a crib for her entire life and had hip dysplasia because of the diaper. The doctors too were concerned, but small bribes were paid to the health authorities to expedite the process. The authorities signed the final set of papers and it was done. Time to go home.

* * *

Greg met them at the airport. He was shocked at how tiny Sophie was. She was hidden in the stroller, covered by a blanket, her head shaking back and forth, her eyes looking down. She never looked at him. They packed her in the car and drove home, speaking little, each lost in their own thoughts. As they turned down their street, all the neighbors came out of their houses to greet the new parents. A large banner was hung on the oak tree of their property: "Welcome home, Sophie!" They drank champagne, congratulated Greg and Marianne, celebrated the arrival of a new child on the street, a playmate for all the children, who were eager to play with Sophie. Only Sophie, at three years of age, could not yet walk, could hardly sit up and roll over, and weighed but fifteen pounds. The neighbors expected to see a cute pudgy baby, cooing, smiling, and responding to adults that ogled her. Instead, Sophie shook, made no eye contact, and steadfastly refused to acknowledge her new neighbors.

Marianne had to learn quickly how to care for the child, who acted like a baby, but was in fact a toddler. The multidisciplinary team at the local child development center was very helpful. They came out to the house and gave Marianne advice on how to stimulate Sophie, how to get her to talk, to handle objects, move her limbs, and so on. Marianne had to learn to change diapers to accommodate her hip dysplasia and to feed Sophie. She could not chew solids, having been fed liquid only, so breakfast could take over an hour. She slept a lot and, when awake, Marianne took her outside in the fresh air. She changed her and fed her according to routine. Greg and Marianne held her close and exercised her limbs. She gained weight, and her motor skills seemed to develop nicely. She stopped shaking, started to hold her head up, sit, and even pulled herself to a standing position.

Soon Sophie went every day to the local child development center for physiotherapy and for the opportunity to interact with other children. Everybody was confident that love, food, and a stimulating environment could bring her out of this predicament. But Sophie did not reward these efforts; she disliked being hugged, she pushed Greg and Marianne away and never looked at them. She never cried for anything even if she were wet, hungry, or cold. To occupy herself she would crawl over to the wall, rock back and forth, and sometimes bang her head against the wall. She would rock in her crib or else pull herself to a standing position and stare at the door without making a sound. Marianne and Greg reasoned to each other that Sophie had chosen to withdraw into her own world. It would take a long time to entice her out of it. As the months went on, she became more and more distant, not less so. She also started to make funny noises. After a full year in treatment, she still was not talking, and her pediatrician wondered whether the deprivation was indeed the cause of her delays in speech and social interaction or whether something else was standing in the way of her progress.

"Did you ever hear the word 'autism'?" her pediatrician asked one day. "I am not saying she is autistic; only that we should consider it as a possibility. Sophie is still not talking and not relating to other people." Marianne knew next to nothing about autism and asked if autism could be caused by the experiences in the orphanage. If so, surely it could be resolved? Love and support could overcome any obstacle, couldn't they?

*   *   *

I was asked to see Sophie at this point to try to determine whether her poor communication skills and her lack of social interaction were due to the deprivation or whether she might have autism. This was a difficult issue to resolve, and it meant sorting out which behavioral characteristics could be explained by living without proper nutrition and stimulation for the first three years of life and which, if any, could be due to autism. Before the appointment, I reviewed the literature on early deprivation and its effect on child development. There were some interesting and informative case reports of children who had experienced terrible deprivation in their formative years. When these children were released from these appalling conditions, they did indeed have many "autistic" characteristics. They were often speech delayed, showed little social interaction, were extremely withdrawn, and demonstrated little capacity for play. However, these autistic-like behaviors attenuated with the provision of a loving environment. It was true that some of the symptoms never completely disappeared. Speech certainly improved, but some of the social oddities persisted. Their social and communication skills seemed to approximate those of younger children, consistent with their overall developmental level. My task was to see if Sophie's social interaction was even more severely delayed than her overall cognitive development. If it was, it would be hard to argue that early deprivation was the only cause of her current difficulties. Social and nutritional deprivation do not cause such uneven development, where some skills are almost age appropriate (like walking and feeding) whereas others (like social–communication) are so delayed.

When I saw Sophie, she was dressed all in red, wore eyeglasses, and darted around the room. She was certainly tiny for her age, and her thick curly brown tresses cascaded onto her shoulders. Her parents carried a bag of sticks and feathers for her to amuse herself with, but instead she preferred to explore the room. She would pick up the toys from the box and look at them briefly but then quickly put them down and turn to something else. She communicated little during our time together but was not eager to leave. I learned from Greg and Marianne that she spoke about six words, but largely had her immediate needs met by placing her parents' hand on a desired object, pointing at things close by, or simply protesting. In most circumstances her parents had to guess what she wanted. She had poor eye contact, smiled only when going for a ride in the taxi to the treatment center, and generally played by herself. She would not ask for help in getting things or to play. She would not share her joy in her play activities, and if her mother was hurt or crying, instead of offering comfort, she would become mad and frustrated. She sometimes sat on her parents' knee during the interview but would not cuddle with them and related only to a few workers who came to the house to work with her. She had no interest in other children at the child development center and would not join in the games. She loved to stare at things. Sophie would bring her eyes right up to a dog's eyes, or to someone wearing glasses or an eye patch. She loved to turn objects like feathers and straws around in her hands. She carried around twigs, Lego blocks, and tree branches. She liked to run in circles and to rock in the car and in front of the TV.

She could also be quite aggressive, although I never saw this during our time together. Sophie was suspended from kindergarten because of this behavior. Apparently she lasted about four days before the teacher and principal started phoning Marianne asking for help. Sometimes they would call as early as 9:15, even before Marianne returned home from dropping her off at school. Her mother was often afraid to leave the house in case she got a call from the teacher saying she had to come and pick her up because she had been aggressive or had hit another child. Eventually Marianne took to not answering the phone so she could take a shower in the morning. More recently, Sophie would have terrible temper tantrums in which she would wail for hours if she were denied an object to hold in her hand, sometimes bite herself, scratch her parents, throw things around the room. These screams felt like a constant reprimand to her parents, a confirmation of their failure to nurture this handicapped little girl.

There was clearly more to Sophie's development than simple developmental delay caused by early deprivation. Sophie was not able to demonstrate the social skills usually seen even in a six-month-old child.

She lacked the motivation to communicate, and her interests were severely restricted, intense, and highly sensory in nature. In addition to the delays caused by the deprivation, I believed she had autism, although it was difficult to sort out which delays in development were due to autism and which due to deprivation. Who knows what neurological damage was caused by the first three years of her life spent in the orphanage? Is it possible for extreme forms of deprivation to cause autism, perhaps in some children who have a genetic risk for the disorder? There are now reports of children from Romanian orphanages presenting with types of autism. It's not inconceivable that in the context of genetic vulnerability the biological insults brought about by lack of food and human touch could be one of the factors causing autism in this child. This is not to say that autism can be caused in the typical circumstance by "bad parenting"; what Sophie experienced was extreme deprivation, malnutrition, and lack of touch, factors known to cause changes in the brain and to influence social behavior in laboratory animals. One cannot generalize from Sophie's history to the vast majority of children with autism in developed countries.

I took a deep breath and tried to explain all this to Greg and Marianne. What I wanted to say was that Sophie did not have autism and that their act of compassion and bravery would be rewarded by a healthy child who would eventually "catch up" if they continued to stimulate and support her. But I knew this was probably not true; the autism was an added burden over and above the early deprivation. Life was going to be even more difficult than they had bargained for during that conversation over the phone. I expected them to be devastated by the news, at the prospect that there would be a limit to Sophie's recovery. In fact, to my surprise, they were relieved. So often my apprehension at communicating bad news turns out to be misguided. Marianne and Greg reasoned that at least Sophie's lack of progress was not due to their failure to love and nurture her. A heavy weight had been lifted. Now at least there was a reason Sophie pushed them away and refused to enter their world. It had a name, and they could get on with the next phase of their lives, dealing with the autism.

*   *   *

I have followed Sophie's progress with interest over the years. Here was an opportunity, I thought, to learn about how parents come to terms with having a child with ASD. The process was all the more dramatic in this family because Greg and Marianne had chosen Sophie out of a sense of compassion. The German poet Rainer Maria Rilke, referring to personal misfortune, wrote to a young friend, "Perhaps everything terrible is, in its deepest being, something helpless that wants nurture from us." The same idea can be applied when an ordinary couple confronts the reality of their child's diagnosis—the challenge is to nourish their misfortune without drowning in it, without being paralyzed by it or denying it. Sometimes the irony of their predicament, that they had chosen Sophie, was too much to bear for Greg and Marianne, but most of the time they were able to accept it without despair, without hopelessness. That acceptance allowed them to move on and to learn from Sophie that even the most vulnerable have hidden gifts. Most families go through this process of acceptance in some fashion, though each family does so in a unique way. But some families search frantically for a cause, for a cure; some become overwhelmed with what to do and end up paralyzed, never able to persevere with a treatment plan that might take months to show results. These are all examples in one form or another of denial, of not accepting the diagnosis, of being resigned to a bleak outcome, something that is avoidable for the most part. Yes, the child has autism; yes, that is a lifelong disability; but no, one does not need to be resigned to an endless wait for some miracle cure or for some cause that can easily be reversed, for someone else to rescue the child from this predicament. There are many interventions that have proven to be helpful, and many of those involve parents working with professionals to facilitate social and communicative development. Above all, acceptance of the diagnosis will call forth from parents a career as forceful advocates for their child, for they will have to advocate with service providers, with teachers, and with members of the community for more services, for better understanding, and for greater inclusion in the community.

How did these parents survive this ordeal? How did they come to their acceptance? Why didn't they give Sophie up? How could they persevere with trying to help her when the situation must have looked so bleak at times? In large part it was because they understood Sophie; they understood where she came from, what she was feeling and thinking, even though she had such limited use of words. They were able to imagine the child behind the autism, see that her preferences and her dislikes were just like those of any child, though admittedly some were a little different. But, like any child, Sophie needed structure and routine, a clear set of expectations, and she needed her parents to be flexible as well. The parameters and expectations for parenting were surely different than one encounters in families with typical children, but the process of parenting was no different. Accepting that Sophie needed to drag that branch to the library, that she needed to look at certain books, and that it did not matter what other people thought about this strange behavior allowed them to appreciate that these behaviors were no reflection on them, on their capacity as parents.

Greg and Marianne learned that sometimes doing nothing was better than frantically doing something. One time Sophie screamed during the night, but they could find no cause. The more they tried to appease her by holding her, rocking her, or distracting her with toys, the worse it got. They just had to let it happen without going into a panic. Once they backed off, and left the room, the upset started to die down, and soon she settled all by herself. They also realized that they had to interpret her simple words as expressing so much more; the word "food" spoken so forcefully sometimes signified a desire for french fries, whereas at other times the same word signified ice cream. Sophie could not be expected to play like other children or communicate about her day. Challenging behavior was to be expected, and the school and other community agencies should be prepared to deal with it without framing it in moral terms.

Greg and Marianne also turned to each other for support and sometimes saw what was funny in Sophie's actions—the love of feathers and twigs, how mother and daughter must have looked walking to the library dragging a branch. They realized what would have happened to Sophie if they had left her in the orphanage. All these insights require a different perspective, an ability to imagine the future, to visualize how others perceive them. It is seeing without prejudice, without metaphors that bind. To support each other, to laugh at themselves, to consider the alternatives all require imagination, an understanding of the other person, whether that person is a spouse, one's community, or one's child's future. Hope was ever present even if fragile and elusive at the end of a long lonely day. Sophie "has climbed more mountains than you will ever see," her mother once said to an unsympathetic school teacher who, in response to challenging behavior at school, offered the opinion that Sophie was spoiled and should be taught some manners. It always surprises me that the people who criticize children with ASD most vehemently are also the ones who appear to lack empathy, are rigid, are resistant to change, and have trouble communicating effectively. There is irony in that too.

Sophie had to learn so much more—to go to stores without fear, to go to school without anxiety. Manners she can probably do without. During those difficult early school years, when Sophie resisted going to school, the mornings were particularly troublesome for Marianne. She had to struggle with Sophie, get her clothes on, encourage her to eat her breakfast and get her out the door to catch the school bus. Often Sophie put up so much resistance that she was late for the bus and Marianne had to drive her to school. Part of the problem was that Marianne felt so much pressure to get things done that much of the morning would be wasted and the many things she had to accomplish that day would be postponed. But once Marianne gave herself time, and the gift of not try-ing to do everything, her sense of pressure decreased and Sophie be-came more compliant. Now she was able to get Sophie off to school in a good mood—a major accomplishment for both of them.

Greg and Marianne have learned to accommodate to Sophie's perspective on the world. They've learned to read her signals and to re-spond to the subtlest forms of nonverbal communication—her grunts, her pointing, her rocking, and her pacing around. These were all indica-tions of some desire or need. Above all they know her routines and her favorite toys, foods, and activities, so they are able to anticipate the meaning of her requests. They sometimes give in to Sophie's demands, recognizing that she has no way to communicate her distress other than by having a temper tantrum, so giving in also teaches Sophie the value of communication. This is all part of Sophie's difficulty in modulating her emotions to the environment. Once her parents understood that, it became easier to tolerate the occasional upheavals. They also learned to see that progress can be measured in small changes that others might overlook. One day she stopped picking up branches on the way to the library. Another day she pointed to a horse in the field while they were driving home. These accomplishments and changes were a great joy to them. These small steps forward were often not visible to others, but her parents could see them and could use them as a buttress against the despair they sometimes felt. They never doubted that Sophie loved them, though she could never communicate that in the traditional way. She would put her arm around her Mom and Dad, stick close to them in unfamiliar and strange environments, sit beside them while watching TV or when she was feeling unwell. If she seemed to reject them at other times, they never doubted that she loved them. She never said "I love you" to them, but of her feelings they had no doubt. They were able to imagine her love and need for them. But most important, they

smiled at her, not only at her eccentricities but also at her courage in going to school even if the teacher was disparaging to her. There were
many embarrassing moments in those early years. Once, Sophie took
her clothes off in the department store. Seeing the looks on the prim
and proper citizens of this small town, eyes riveted at this spectacle of a
naked girl running up and down the aisles, brought smiles to their
faces. At the time, they were quite upset to be sure, but time gives perspective and with perspective comes the distance to be amused.

Sophie improved slowly with time. Although she is still largely
nonverbal, she has shown more motivation to communicate using signs
and a picture exchange system, and she seems to understand more. She
still loves feathers and sticks and loves to fit things together, such as
pencils and springs. She also likes to paint with feathers and to look at
books. Sophie will not go to the bathroom without a book about the
Simpsons. She loves Maggie, the baby, because of the frequent tears she
sheds. Sophie enjoys listening to her parents' old rock and roll records
from the '70s, especially the Woodstock album. She plays some chords
on the piano and will sit through an entire church service as long as she
is allowed to play the piano at the end. She likes to be with people, especially adults in her extended family. She likes to touch others and to
put her arm around her mother's waist, although she still does not like
to be touched herself. Her mother says, "She is a very loving child in her
own way." It's the "in her own way" that marks the process of acceptance without resignation. Her parents can read these behaviors as expressions of love, even though they might not be recognized as such by
others. And it doesn't matter. The ability to see behavior not tradition-
ally associated with feelings of love but being able to imagine, to discern
its purpose in this context, is what is important. This is what leads to a
sense of hope that avoids resignation and despair. There is meaning in
these behaviors—there is a communication, a language—if only the
code can be broken. These parents were able to break that code once
they accepted that there was a different language.

Just the other day, Sophie participated in drama class. She pre-
tended to be a baby-sitter looking after a crying infant. She fed the doll,
cuddled her, and wrapped her in a blanket. She made the teacher and
her classmates smile as they could recognize that this was something
new and special. When she was done, they all clapped their hands enthusiastically in appreciation. Sophie beamed with delight and wanted
to stay on the makeshift "stage." Her new teacher had to lead her off to
let someone else have a turn but wrote about this story with great en-

thusiasm in the report she sent home to Sophie's parents. Marianne and Greg were delighted for days and made a special point of telling me.

* * *

If this were a fairy tale, the story should have a "happy" ending. The act of bravery, courage, and compassion should be rewarded with the emergence of a normal child who plays with the other children on the street, who goes to her local school and to fast food outlets to eat hamburgers and french fries. But no, instead she draws pictures with feathers, drags a branch along the ground, and is silent. But this *is* a happy ending. Sophie is no disappointment to her parents. They do not for one moment regret the fateful decision to adopt her. That one choice was made in an instant, in full knowledge of its consequences for them, if not for her.

Each family of a child with autism has its own defining moment, and in point of fact there are many such moments in a family's lifetime. Moments when a decision is made, when a realization happens, when the past with its naive hopes and dreams is let go and a future is chosen, accepted with equanimity, repose, and resolve. Sometimes that moment first occurs when a diagnosis is given, sometimes it first occurs after many years when the expected cure or recovery does not materialize. That defining moment is an acceptance of the weight of biological fate but not a surrender to its limits. Each family eventually realizes what life has in store for them and can accept that but will never give up the struggle to improve the lot of their child and to advocate for more and better services for all children. The act of rescue performed by Greg and Marianne was such a defining act, made very early on by two people in the silence of their own hearts, over the telephone thousands of miles apart. They had the courage to choose this misfortune, they took it in, nourished it, then challenged and celebrated it. In the process, they themselves were transformed. By taking small steps every day and learning Sophie's secret language, they learned the value of seeing with new perspectives, of imagining the mind of their child, so dark and mysterious, and of seeing the gifts within the disability. Sophie gave them the courage to achieve a state of compassion, which is as close to grace as possible nowadays. Courage does indeed lie in small acts performed every day by ordinary people who find themselves in unexpected circumstances. Others might say such acts are foolish, but then foolishness is often the prerogative of the brave.

In a sense all children with autism come from an orphanage, because they are foreign to us. The choice Marianne and Greg had to make in that apartment in Bucharest, all parents have to make when they decide to accept the inevitability of the diagnosis, when they realize that their future will not be what they planned, when they give up searching for a cause, when they stop searching for the perfect cure. Each of those moments is a defining act; it takes courage and the capacity to laugh at the irony of the presumption that plans can be made, that life follows a predictable course like a river, that it has a direction and a meaning, other than the one of getting through this day to the next, of getting Sophie off to school in a good mood.

Bibliography

CHAPTER 1

American Psychiatric Association. (1994). *Diagnostic and statistical manual of mental disorders* (4th ed.). Washington: American Psychiatric Association.

Chakrabarti, S., & Fombonne, E. (2001). Pervasive developmental disorders in preschool children. *Journal of the American Medical Association, 285,* 3093–3099.

Kanner, L. (1973). *Childhood psychosis: Initial studies and new insights.* Washington, DC: Winston.

Kolvin, I., Ounsted, C., & Roth, M. (1971). Studies in the childhood psychoses. V. Cerebral dysfunction and childhood psychoses. *British Journal of Psychiatry, 118*(545), 407–414.

Mahoney, W. J., Szatmari, P., MacLean, J. E., Bryson, S. E., Bartolucci, G., Walter, S. D., Jones, M. B., & Zwaigenbaum, L. (1998). Reliability and accuracy of differentiating pervasive developmental disorder subtypes. *Journal of the American Academy of Child and Adolescent Psychiatry, 37*(3), 278–285.

Rutter, M. (1968). Concepts of autism: A review of research. *Journal of Child Psychology and Psychiatry, 9*(1), 1–25.

Sontag, S. (1990). *Illness as metaphor and AIDS and its metaphor.* New York: Doubleday.

Szatmari, P., Archer, L., Fisman, S., Streiner, D. L., & Wilson, F. (1995). Asperger's syndrome and autism: Differences in behavior, cognition and adaptive functioning. *Journal of the American Academy of Child and Adolescent Psychiatry, 34*(12), 1662–1671.

Szatmari, P., Bryson, S. E., Streiner, D. L., Wilson, F., Archer, L., & Ryers, C. (2000). Two-year outcome of preschool children with autism or Asperger's syndrome. *American Journal of Psychiatry, 157*(12), 1980–1987.

Tanguay, P. E. (2000). Pervasive developmental disorders: A 10-year review. *Jour-*

nal of the American Academy of Child and Adolescent Psychiatry, 39(9), 1079–1095.

Wing, L. (1988). The continuum of autistic characteristics. In E. Schopler & G. B. Mesibov (Eds.), *Diagnosis and assessment in autism* (pp. 91–110). New York: Plenum Press.

CHAPTER 2

Barron, J., & Barron, S. (1992). *There's a boy in here*. New York: Simon & Schuster.

Chin, H. Y., & Bernard-Opitz, V. (2000). Teaching conversational skills to children with autism: Effect on the development of a theory of mind. *Journal of Autism and Developmental Disorders, 30*(6), 569–583.

Happe, F. (1999). Autism: Cognitive deficit or cognitive style? *Trends in Cognitive Science, 3*(6), 216–222.

Kephart, B. (1998). *A slant of sun: One child's courage*. New York: Norton.

National Research Council. (2001). *Educating children with autism*. Washington, DC: National Academy Press.

CHAPTER 3

Baron-Cohen, S., Ring, H. A., Bullmore, E. T., Wheelwright, S., Ashwin, C., & Williams, S. C. (2000). The amygdala theory of autism. *Neuroscience and Behavioural Reviews, 24*, 355–364.

Brian, J. A., Tipper, S. P., Weaver, B., & Bryson, S. E.(2003). Inhibitory mechanisms in autism spectrum disorders: Typical selective inhibition of location versus facilitated perceptual processing. *Journal of Child Psychology and Psychiatry, 44*(4), 552–560.

Frith, U. (1996). Cognitive explanations of autism. *Acta Paediatrica Supplement, 416*, 63–68.

Happe, F., & Frith, U. (1996). The neuropsychology of autism. *Brain, 119*(Pt. 4), 1377–1400.

Hermelin, B., Pring, L., & Heavey, L. (1994). Visual and motor functions in graphically gifted savants. *Psychological Medicine, 24*(3), 673–680.

Hollander, E. (1998). Treatment of obsessive-compulsive spectrum disorders with SSRIs. *British Journal of Psychiatry* (Suppl. 35), 7–12.

Jolliffe, T., & Baron-Cohen, S. (1997). Are people with autism and Asperger syndrome faster than normal on the Embedded Figures Test? *Journal of Child Psychology and Psychiatry, 38*(5), 527–534.

McDougle, C. J., Naylor, S. T., Cohen, D. J., Volkmar, F. R., Heninger, G. R., & Price, L. H. (1996). A double-blind, placebo-conrolled study of fluvoxamine in adults with autism disorder. *Archives of General Psychiatry, 53*(11), 1001–1008.

Oe, K. (1986). *Rouse up o young men of the new age.* New York: Grove Press.

Russell, J. (Ed.). (1997). *Autism as an executive disorder.* New York: Oxford University Press.

Siegal, M., & Varley, R. (2002). Neural systems involved in "theory of mind." *Nature Reviews, Neuroscience, 3*(6), 463–471.

Tredgold, A. F. (1937). *A text-book of mental deficiency.* Baltimore: Wood.

Wainwright-Sharp, J. A., & Bryson, S. E. (1993). Visual orienting deficits in high-functioning people with autism. *Journal of Autism and Developmental Disorders, 23*(1), 1–13.

CHAPTER 4

Bryan, L. C., & Gast, D. L. (2000). Teaching on-task and on-schedule behaviors to high-functioning children with autism via picture activity schedules. *Journal of Autism and Developmental Disorders, 30*(6), 553–567.

CHAPTER 5

Baron-Cohen, S. (1989). The autistic child's theory of mind: A case of specific developmental delay. *Journal of Child Psychology and Psychiatry, 30*(2), 285–297.

Baron-Cohen, S., Wheelwright, S., Hill J., Raste, Y., & Plumb, I. (2001). The "Reading the Mind in the Eyes" Test revised version: A study with normal adults, and adults with Asperger syndrome or high-functioning autism. *Journal of Child Psychology and Psychiatry, 42*(2), 241–251.

Carruthers, P., & Smith, P. K. (Eds.). (1996). *Theories of theories of mind.* Cambridge, UK: Cambridge University Press.

Gerland, G., & Tate, J. (2003). *A real person: Life on the outside.* London: Souvenir Press.

Ozonoff, S., & Miller, J. N. (1995). Teaching theory of mind: a new approach to social skills training for individuals with autism. *Journal of Autism and Developmental Disorders, 25*(4), 415–433.

Rutherford, M. D., Baron-Cohen, S., & Wheelwright, S. (2002). Reading the mind in the voice: A study with normal adults and adults with Asperger syndrome and high functioning autism. *Journal of Autism and Developmental Disorders, 32*(3), 189–194.

Thiemann, K. S., & Goldstein, H. (2001). Social stories, written text cues and video feedback: Effects on social communication of children with autism. *Journal of Applied Behavior Analysis, 34*(4), 425–446.

Williams, D. (1995). *Somebody somewhere: Breaking free from the world of autism.* New York: Three Rivers Press.

Yirmiya, N., Erel, O., Shaked, M., & Solomonica-Levi, D. (1998). Meta-analyses comparing theory of mind abilities of individuals with autism, individuals with mental retardation, and normally developing individuals. *Psychological Bulletin, 124*(3), 283–307.

Yirmiya, N., Solomonica-Levi, D., Shulman, C., & Pilowsky, T. (1996). Theory of mind abilities in individuals with autism, Down syndrome, and mental retardation of unknown etiology: The role of age and intelligence. *Journal of Child Psychology and Psychiatry, 37*(8), 1003–1013.

CHAPTER 6

Bottini, G., Corcoran, R., Sterzi, R., Paulesu, E., Schenone, P., Scarpa, P., Frackowiak, R. S., & Frith C. D. (1994). The role of the right hemisphere in the interpretation of figurative aspects of language: A positron emission tomography activation study. *Brain, 117*, 1241–1253.

Faust, M., & Weisper, S. (2000). Understanding metaphoric sentences in the two cerebral hemispheres. *Brain and Cognition, 43*(1–3), 186–191.

Fine, J., Bartolucci, G., Ginsberg, G., & Szatmari P. (1991). The use of intonation to communicate in pervasive developmental disorders. *Journal of Child Psychology and Psychiatry, 32*(5), 771–782.

Fine, J., Bartolucci, G., Szatmari, P., & Ginsberg, G. (1994). Cohesive discourse in pervasive developmental disorders. *Journal of Autism and Developmental Disorders, 24*(3), 315–329.

Frith, U., & Happe, F. (1994). Language and communication in autistic disorders. *Philosophical Transactions of the Royal Society of London, Series B, Biological Sciences, 346*(1315), 97–104.

Goldstein, H. (2002). Communication intervention for children with autism: A review of treatment efficacy. *Journal of Autism and Developmental Disorders, 32*(5), 373–396.

Happe, F. G. (1993). Communicative competence and theory of mind in autism: a test of relevance theory. *Cognition, 48*(2), 101–119.

Keen, D., Sigafoos, J., & Woodyatt, G. (2001). Replacing prelinguistic behaviors with functional communication. *Journal of Autism and Developmental Disorders, 31*(4), 385–98.

Kircher, T. T., Brammer, M., Tous Andreu, N., Williams, S. C., & McGuire, P. K. (2001). Engagement of right temporal cortex during processing of linguistic context. *Neuropsychologia, 39*(8), 798–809.

Koegel, L. K.(2000). Interventions to facilitate communication in autism. *Journal of Autism and Developmental Disorders, 30*(5), 383–391.

Lord, C. (2000). Commentary: Achievements and future directions for intervention research in communication and autism spectrum disorders. *Journal of Autism and Developmental Disorders, 30*(5), 393–398.

Loveland, K. A., & Tunali, B. (1991). Social scripts for conversational interactions in autism and Down syndrome. *Journal of Autism and Developmental Disorders, 21*(2), 177–186.

CHAPTER 7

Kanner, L. (1971). Follow-up study of eleven autistic children originally reported in 1943. *Journal of Autism and Child Schizopzhrenia, 1*(2), 119–145.
Kanner, L., Rodriguez, A., & Aschenden, B. (1972). How far can autistic children go in matters of social adaptation? *Journal of Autism and Child Schizophrenia,* 2(1), 9–33.
Nordin, V., & Gillberg, C. (1998). The long-term course of autistic disorders: Update on follow-up studies. *Acta Psychiatrica Scandinavica, 97*(2), 99–108.

CHAPTER 8

Carrey, N. J. (1995). Itard's 1828 memoire on "Mutism caused by a lesion of the intellectual functions": A historical analysis. *Journal of the American Academy of Child and Adolescent Psychiatry, 34*(12), 1655–1661.
Croen, L. A., Grether, J. K., Hoogstrate, J., & Selvin, S. (2002). The changing prevalence of autism in California. *Journal of Autism and Developmental Disorders, 32*(3), 207–215.
Gurney, J. G., Fritz, M. S., Ness, K. K., Sievers, P., Newschaffer, C. J., & Shapiro, E. G. (2003). Analysis of prevalence trends of autism spectrum disorder in Minnesota. *Archives of Pediatrics and Adolescent Medicine, 157*(7), 622–627.
Szatmari, P. (2003). The causes of autism spectrum disorders. *British Medical Journal, 326*(7382), 173–174.

CHAPTER 9

Bibby, P., Eikeseth, S., Martin, N. T., Mudford, O. C., & Reeves, D. (2002). Progress and outcomes for children with autism receiving parent-managed intensive interventions. *Research in Developmental Disabilities, 22*(6), 425–447.
Bondy, A. S., & Frost, L. A. (1998). The picture exchange communication system. *Seminars in Speech and Language, 19*(4), 373–388.
Boyd, R. D., & Corley, M. J. (2001). Outcome survey of early intensive behavioural intervention for young children with autism in a community setting. *Autism, 5*(4), 430–441.
Charlop-Christy, M. H., Carpenter, M., Le, L., LeBlanc, L. A., & Kellet, K. (2002). Using the picture exchange communication system (PECS) with children with autism: Assessment of PECS acquisition, speech, social-communica-

tive behavior, and problem behavior. *Journal of Applied Behavior Analysis*, 35(3), 213–231.

Charman, T., Howlin, P., Aldred, C., Baird, G., Degli Espinosa, F., Diggle, T., Kovshoff, H., Law, J., Le Courteur, A., MacNiven, J., Magiati, I., Martin, N., McConachie, H., Peacock, S., Pickles, A., Randle, V., Slonims, V., & Wolke, D. (2003). Research into early intervention for children with autism and related disorders: Methodological and design issues. *Autism*, 7(2), 217–225.

Diggle, T., McConachie, H. R., & Randle, V. R. (2003). Parent-mediated early intervention for young children with autism spectrum disorder. *Cochrane Database of Systematic Reviews*, (1)CD003496.

Drew, A., Baird, G., Baron-Cohen, S., Cox, A., Slonims, V., Wheelwright, S., Swettenham, J., Berry, B., & Charman, T. (2002). A pilot randomized control trial of a parent training intervention for preschool children with autism: Preliminary findings and methodological challenges. *European Child and Adolescent Psychiatry*, 11(6), 266–272.

Harris, S. L., & Handleman, J. S. (2000). Age and IQ at intake as predictors of placement for young children with autism: A four-to six-year follow-up. *Journal of Autism and Developmental Disorders*, 30(2), 137–142.

Hastings, R. P., & Symes, M. D. (2002). Early intensive behavioural intervention for children with autism: Parental therapeutic self-efficacy. *Research in Developmental Disabilities*, 23(5), 332–341.

Kravits, T. R., Kamps, D. M., Kemmerer, K., & Potucek, J. (2002). Brief report: Increasing communication skills for an elementary-aged student with autism using the Picture Exchange Communication System. *Journal of Autism and Developmental Disorders*, 32(3), 225–230.

Lauchey, K. M., & Heflin, L. J. (2000). Enhancing social skills of kindergarten children with autism through the training of multiple peers as tutors. *Journal of Autism and Developmental Disorders*, 30(3), 183–193.

McConnell, S. R. (2002). Interventions to facilitate social interaction for young children with autism: review of available research and recommendations for educational interventions and future research. *Journal of Autism and Developmental Disorders*, 32(5), 351–372.

Pierce, K., & Schreibman, L. (1997). Multiple peer use of pivotal response training to increase social behaviors of classmates with autism: Results from trained and untrained peers. *Journal of Applied Behavior Analysis*, 30(1), 157–160.

Salt, J., Sellars, V., Shemilt, J., Boyd, S., Couson, T., & McCool, S. (2001). The Scottish Centre for Autism preschool treatment programme. I: A developmental approach to early intervention. *Autism*, 5(4), 362–373.

Sheinkopf, S. J., & Siegel, B. (1998). Home-based behavioural treatment of young children with autism. *Journal of Autism and Developmental Disorders*, 28(1), 15–23.

Smith, T., Groen, A. D., & Wynn, J. W. (2000). Randomized trial of intensive early intervention for children with pervasive developmental disorder. *American Journal of Mental Retardation, 105*(4), 269–285.

CHAPTER 10

Goldstein, H., & Cisar, C. L. (1992). Promoting interaction during sociodramatic play: Teaching scripts to typical preschoolers and classmates with disabilities. *Journal of Applied Behavioral Analysis, 25*(2), 265–280.

Harrower, J. K, & Dunlap, G. (2001). Including children with autism in general education classrooms: A review of effective strategies. *Behavior Modification, 25*(5), 762–784.

Horner, R. H., Carr, E. G., Strain, P. S., Todd, A. W., & Reed, H. K. (2002). Problem behavior interventions for young children with autism: A research synthesis. *Journal of Autism and Developmental Disorders, 32*(5), 423–446.

Kasari, C., Freeman, S. F., Bauminger, N., & Alkin, M. C. (1999). Parental perspectives on inclusion: Effects of autism and Down syndrome. *Journal of Autism and Developmental Disorders, 1999, 29*(4), 297–305.

Krantz, P. J., & McClannahan, L. E. (1998). Social interaction skills for children with autism: A script-fading procedure for beginning readers. *Journal of Applied Behavior Analysis, 31*(2), 191–202.

McDougle, C. J., Stigler, K. A., & Posey, D. J. (2003). Treatment of aggression in children and adolescents with autism and conduct disorder. *Journal of Clinical Psychiatry, 4*, 16–25.

McGregor, E., & Campbell, E. (2001). The attitudes of teachers in Scotland to the integration of children with autism into mainstream schools. *Autism, 5*(2), 189–207.

Robertson, K., Chamberlain, B., & Kasari, C. (2003). General education teachers' relationships with included students with autism. *Journal of Autism and Developmental Disorders, 33*(2), 123–130.

Roeyers, H. (1996). The influence of nonhandicapped peers on the social interactions of children with a pervasive developmental disorder. *Journal of Autism and Developmental Disorders, 26*(3), 303–320.

Turnbull, H. R., III, Wilcox, B. L., & Stowe, M. J. (2002). A brief overview of special education law with a focus on autism. *Journal of Autism and Developmental Disorders, 32*(5), 479–493.

Weiss, M. J., & Harris, S. L. (2001). Teaching social skills to people with autism. *Behavior Modification, 25*(5), 785–802.

CHAPTER 11

Borges, J. L. (1967). *A personal anthology.* New York: Grove Weidenfeld.

Chen, S. H., & Bernard-Opitz, G. (1993). Comparison of personal and computer-assisted instruction for children with autism. *Mental Retardation, 31*(6), 368–376.

Ehlers, S., Nyden, A., Gillberg, C., Sandberg, A. D., Dahlgren, S. O., Hjelmquist, E., & Oden, A. (1997). Asperger syndrome, autism and attention disorders: A comparative study of cognitive profiles of 120 children. *Journal of Child Psychology and Psychiatry, 38*(2), 207–217.

Goldstein, G., Beers, S. R., Siegel, D. J., & Minshew, N. J. (2001). A comparison of WAIS-R profiles in adults with high-functioning autism and differing subtypes of learning disability. *Applied Neuropsychology, 8*(3), 148–154.

Goldstein, G., Siegel, D. J, & Minshew, N. J. (1995). Abstraction and problem solving in autism: Further categorization of the fundamental deficit. *Archives in Clinical Neuropsychology, 10*(4), 335.

Heimann, M., Nelson, K. E., Tjus, T., & Gillberg, C. (1995). Increasing reading and communication skills in children with autism through an intervactive multimedia computer program. *Journal of Autism and Developmental Disorders, 25*(5), 459–480.

Joseph, R. M., Tager-Flusberg, H., & Lord, C. (2002). Cognitive profiles and social-communicative functioning in children with autism spectrum disorder. *Journal of Child Psychology and Psychiatry, 43*(6), 807–821.

Klin, A., Volkmar, F. R., Sparrow, S. S., Cicchetti, D. V., & Rourke, B. P. (1995). Validity and neuropsychological characterization of Asperger syndrome: Convergence with nonverbal learning disabilities syndrome. *Journal of Child Psychology and Psychiatry, 36*(7), 1127–1140.

McDonald, B. C. (2002). Recent developments in the application of the nonverbal learning disabilities model. *Current Psychiatry Reports, 4*(5), 323–330.

Minshew, N. J., Meyer, J., & Goldstein, G. (2002). Abstract reasoning in autism: A dissociation between concept formation and concept identification. *Neuropsychology, 16*(3), 327–234.

Minshew, N. J., Siegel, D. J., Goldstein, G., & Weldy, S. (1994). Verbal problem solving in high functioning autistic individuals. *Archives in Clinical Neuropsychology, 9*(1), 31–40.

Moore, M., & Calvert, S. (2000). Brief report: Vocabulary acquisition for children with autism: teacher or computer instruction. *Journal of Autism and Developmental Disorders, 30*(4), 359–362.

Szatmari, P., Tuff, L., Finlayson, M. A., & Bartolucci, G. (1990). Asperger's syndrome and autism: Neurocognitive aspects. *Journal of the American Academy of Child and Adolescent Psychiatry, 29*(1), 130–136.

Tager-Flusberg, H., & Joseph, R. M. (2003). Identifying neurocognitive phenotypes in autism. *Philosophical Transactions of the Royal Society of London, Series B, Biological Sciences, 358*(1430), 303–314.

Williams, C., Wright, B., Callaghan, G., & Coughlan, B. (2002). Do children with autism learn to read more readily by computer assisted instruction or traditional book methods? A pilot study. *Autism, 6*(1), 71–91.

CHAPTER 12

Rutter, M., Andersen-Wood, L., Beckett, C., Bredenkamp, D. Castle, J., Groothues, C., Kreppner, J., Keaveney, L., Lord, C., & O'Connor, T. G. (1999). Quasi-autistic patterns following severe early global privation: English and Romanian Adoptees (ERA) Study Team. *Journal of Child Psychology and Psychiatry, 40*(4), 537–549.

Resources

WEBSITES

Autism Society Canada

ASC was founded in 1976 by a group of parents to encourage the formation of autism societies and to address national autism issues. Today, ASC is the only national autism charitable organization committed to advocacy, public education, information and referral, and provincial development support.

Autism Society of Canada
P.O. Box 65
Orangeville, Ontario, Canada L9W 2Z5
Phone: 519-942-8720
Fax: 519- 942-3566
Toll Free: 1-866-874-3334
E-mail: *info@autismsocietycanada.ca*
Website: *www.autismsocietycanada.ca*

The Source: Autism, Asperger Syndrome, Pervasive Developmental Disorders, MAAP Services (Asperger Syndrome Coalition of the United States has joined forces with MAAP Services for Autism and Asperger Syndrome)

MAAP Services for the Autism Spectrum is a nonprofit organization dedicated to providing information and advice to families of more advanced (higher-functioning) individuals with autism, Asperger syndrome, and pervasive developmental disorder (PDD).

MAAP Services, Inc.
P.O. Box 524
Crown Point, IN 46307

Phone: 219-662-1311
Fax: 219-662-0638
E-mail: *chart@netnitco.net*
Website: www.maapservices.org

Autism Society of America

The Autism Society of America was founded in 1965 by a small group of parents working on a volunteer basis out of their homes. Over the last 35 years, the society has developed into the leading source of information and referral on autism. Today, over 20,000 members are connected through a working network of over 200 chapters in nearly every state.

Autism Society of America
7910 Woodmont Avenue, Suite 300
Bethesda, MD 20814-3067
Phone: 301-657-0881 or 1-800-3AUTISM
E-mail: *info@autism-society.org*
Website: *www.autism-societiy.org*

CanChild Centre for Childhood Disability Research

CanChild is comprised of a multidisciplinary team working in the field of childhood disability. Research programs at CanChild concentrate on children and youth with disabilities and their families.

CanChild Centre for Childhood Disability Research
Institute for Applied Health Sciences
McMaster University
1400 Main Street West, Room 408
Hamilton, Ontario, Canada L8S 1C7
Phone: 905-525-9140, ext. 27850
Fax: 905-522-6095
E-mail: *canchild@mcmaster.ca*
Website: *www.fhs.mcmaster.ca/canchild*

Exploring Autism

Up-to-date information on genetic research into autism.

Website: *www.exploringautism.org*

National Autistic Society (UK)

The National Autistic Society (NAS) is registered both with the Charity Commissioners and the Registrar of Companies. The charity's objective is to provide education, treatment, welfare and care to people with autism and related conditions.

NAS Scotland
Central Chambers
109 Hope Street, 1st Floor
Glasgow, Scotland G2 6LL
Tel: +44-0-141-221-8090
Fax: +44-0-141-221-8118
E-mail: *scotland@nas.org.uk*
Website: *www.nas.org.uk*

OASIS - Online Asperger Syndrome Information and Support

This is an organization for families of children diagnosed with Asperger syndrome and related disorders, educators who teach children with Asperger syndrome, professionals working with individuals diagnosed with Asperger syndrome, and individuals with Asperger syndrome who are seeking support to have access to information.

E-mail: *bkirby@udel.edu*
Website: *www.udel.edu.bkirby/asperger*

ASPEN - Asperger Syndrome Professional Network (UK)

ASPEN is a group of professionals involved in developing services for children and adults with Asperger syndrome.

Asperger Syndrome Professional Network
National Autistic Society
Castle Heights
72 Maid Marian Way, 4th Floor
Nottingham, United Kingdom
NG1 6BJ
Phone: 0-115-911-3360
E-mail: *abicknell@nas.org.uk*
Website: *www.nas.org.uk/profs/aspen*

BIOME

BIOME is a collection of gateways that provide access to evaluated, quality Internet resources in the health and life sciences, aimed at students, researchers, academics, and practitioners. BIOME is created by a core team of information specialists and subject experts based at the University of Nottingham Greenfield Medical Library.

BIOME
Greenfield Medical Library
Queens Medical Centre
Nottingham, United Kingdom

NG7 2UH
E-mail: *help@biome.ac.uk*
Website: *www.biome.ac.uk*

National Alliance for Autism Research

NAAR is the first organization in the United States dedicated to funding and accelerating biomedical research focusing on autism spectrum disorders.

National Office, NAAR
99 Wall Street, Research Park
Princeton, NJ 08540
Phone: 888-777-NAAR
Fax: 609-430-9163
Website: *www.naar.org*

National Institute of Mental Health (US) - Autism page

National Institute of Mental Health (NIMH)
Office of Communications
6001 Executive Boulevard, Room 8184, MSC 9663
Bethesda, MD 20892-9663
Phone: 301-443-4513 or 1-866-615-NIMH (6464), toll-free
TTY: 301-443-8431; Fax: 301-443-4279
Fax 4U: 301-443-5158
E-mail: *nimhinfo@nih.gov*
Website: *www.nimh.nih.gov/publicat/autismmenu.cfm*

PsychDirect

The public education site of the Department of Psychiatry and Behavioural Neuroscience of McMaster University contains the author's research page (click on "Autism" under "Children's Issues" on the home page), which describes the studies currently under way but also provides an autism glossary, a newsletter, FAQs and facts versus myths, a list of the autism societies and support groups across Canada, and links to other valuable resources.

Website: *www.psychdirect.com*

BOOKS

Attwood, T. (1998). *Asperger's syndrome: A guide for parents and professionals.* London: Jessica Kingsley.
Baron-Cohen, S. (1995). *Mindblindness: An essay on autism and theory of mind.* Cambridge, MA: MIT Press.

Faherty, C., & Mesibov, G. B. (2000). *Asperger's: What does it mean to me?* Arlington, TX: Future Horizons.

Frith, U. (1992). *Autism: Explaining the enigma.* Malden, MA: Blackwell.

Fouse, B., & Wheeler, M. (1997). *A treasure chest of behavioral strategies for individuals with autism.* Arlington, TX: Future Horizons.

Grandin, T. (1986). *Emergence: Labeled autistic.* Novato, CA: Academic Therapy Publications.

Grandin, T. (1996). *Thinking in pictures: And other reports from my life with autism.* New York: Vintage Books.

Gray, C. (2000). *The new social story book: Illustrated edition.* Arlington, TX: Future Horizons.

Harris, S. L. (2003). *Right from the start: Behavioral intervention for young children with autism: A guide for parents and professionals.* Bethesda, MD: Woodbine House.

Harris, S. L. (2003). *Siblings of children with autism: A guide for families* (2nd ed.). Bethesda, MD: Woodbine House.

Hogdon, L. A. (1999). *Solving behavior problems in autism.* Troy, MI: QuirkRoberts Publishing.

Hogdon, L. A. (1995). *Visual strategies for improving communication: Practical supports for school and home.* Troy, MI: QuirkRoberts Publishing.

Howlin, P. (1997). *Autism: Preparing for adulthood.* New York: Routledge: New York.

Howlin, P. (1998). *Behavioural approaches to problems in childhood.* London: Mac Keith Press.

Howlin, P., Baron-Cohen, S., & Hadwin, J. (1998). *Teaching children with autism to mind-read: A practical guide for teachers and parents.* Indianapolis, IN: Wiley.

Lynn, E., & McClannahan, P. J. (2003). *Activity schedules for children with autism: Teaching independent behavior.* Bethesda, MD: Woodbine House.

Maurice, C. (1996). *Behavioral intervention for young children with autism: A manual for parents and professionals.* Austin, TX: Pro-Ed.

Ozonoff, S., Dawson, G., & McPartland, J. (2002). *A parent's guide to Asperger syndrome and high-functioning autism: How to meet the challenges and help your child thrive.* New York: Guilford Press.

Quill, K. A. (2000). *Do-watch-listen-say: Social and communication intervention for children with autism.* Baltimore: Brookes.

Romanowski Bashe, P., & Kirby, B. L. (2001). *The oasis guide to Asperger syndrome: Advice, support, insights and inspiration.* New York: Crown.

Siegel, B. (1996). *The world of the autistic child: Understanding and treating autistic spectrum disorders.* London: Oxford University Press.

Weiss, M. J., & Harris, S. L. (2001). *Reaching out, joining in: Teaching social skills to young children with autism.* Bethesda, MD: Woodbine House.

Wetherby, A. M., & Prizant, B. M. (Eds.). (2000). *Autism spectrum disorders: A transactional developmental perspective.* Baltimore: Brookes.

Index

About the Author

Peter Szatmari, MD, has been working in the field of autism and pervasive developmental disorders for more than twenty years. He is the director of the Canadian Autism Intervention Research Network (CAIRN), a group of parents, clinicians, and scientists attempting to develop a research agenda on early intervention in autism. CAIRN supports a website (*www.cairn-site.com*) that disseminates the latest evidence-based information on early intervention and screening in autism.

Dr. Szatmari is supported by a Senior Research Fellowship Award from the Ontario Mental Health Foundation and is editor of the journal *Evidence-Based Mental Health*. He was instrumental in developing the Pervasive Developmental Disorder Team at Chedoke Child and Family Centre, a regional diagnostic and treatment program for children with this diagnosis. He served for five years on the Board of Directors of Autism Society Ontario and as the chairman of the Research Committee for that organization. He has been a consultant to various government agencies in Canada, the United States, and internationally on research and on treatment services for children with autism spectrum disorders.

Currently, Dr. Szatmari is Professor of Psychiatry and Behavioral Neurosciences, Vice-Chair of Research, and Head of the Division of Child Psychiatry at McMaster University. He is also a member of the Offord Centre for Child Studies and holds the Chedoke Health Chair in Child Psychiatry at McMaster University.